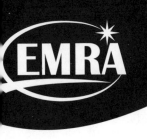

Emergency Medicine
Advocacy
HANDBOOK
3rd Edition

Nathaniel R. Schlicher, MD, JD, FACEP
Alison Haddock, MD
Editors-in-Chief

D1515951

EMERGENCY MEDICINE RESIDENTS' ASSOCIATION

Disclaimer

The Emergency Medicine Residents' Association makes every effort to ensure that contributors to EMRA-sponsored publications are knowledgeable authorities in their fields. Readers are nevertheless advised that the statements and opinions expressed in this book are provided as guidelines and should not be construed as EMRA policy unless specifically referred to as such. EMRA disclaims any liability or responsibility of the consequences or any actions taken in reliance on those statements or opinions. The materials contained herein are not intended to establish policy or procedure.

Emergency Medicine Residents' Association
1125 Executive Circle
Irving, TX 75038-2522
972-550-0920
www.emra.org

Please send comments or suggestions to emra@emra.org.

2013 Advocacy Handbook
Editorial Staff

Editors-in-Chief

Nathaniel R. Schlicher, MD, JD, FACEP
Former EMRA Legislative Advisor (2008-2010)
Associate Director, TeamHealth Patient Safety Organization

Alison Haddock, MD
Former EMRA Legislative Advisor (2010-2012)
Attending Emergency Physician

Chapter Authors

Kevin Blythe
EMRA MSC Legislative Coordinator,
2012-2013
Meharry Medical College
Fourth-Year Medical Student

Kene A. Chukwuanu, MD
EMRA Membership Development Coordinator,
2012-2014
Saint Louis University School of Medicine
Emergency Medicine Resident

Jordan Celeste, MD
EMRA President-Elect, 2012-2013
Brown University
Emergency Medicine Resident

Robert Cooper, MD, MPH
The Wexner Medical Center at
Ohio State University
Emergency Medicine Chief Resident

Eric Cortez, MD
The Wexner Medical Center at
Ohio State University
Emergency Medicine Chief Resident

Cameron A. Decker, MD
EMRA President, 2012-2013
Baylor College of Medicine
Emergency Medicine Resident

Nathan Deal, MD
Former EMRA President
(2010-2011)
Baylor College of Medicine
Attending Emergency Physician
and Assistant Professor

Ramnik S. Dhaliwal, MD, JD
Hennepin County Medical Center
Emergency Medicine/Internal Medicine
Resident

Brooke L. Donaldson, MD
Akron General Medical Center and Northeast
Ohio Medical University
Emergency Medicine Resident

Michael Dorrity, MD
Attending Emergency Physician

Kael Duprey, MD, JD
North Shore-Long Island Jewish
Emergency Medicine Resident

Zachary Ginsberg, MD, MPP
North Shore University Hospital
Emergency Medicine Resident

Puneet Gupta, MD
EMRA Health Policy Committee,
Vice-Chair, 2012-2013
Central Michigan University
Emergency Medicine Resident

Lindsay M. Harmon-Hardin, MD
Indiana University
Attending Emergency Physician

Sarah Hoper, MD, JD
EMRA Legislative Advisor,
2012-2014
Washington University in St. Louis
Emergency Medicine Resident

continued

Dennis Hsieh, MD, JD
Alameda County Medical Center/
Highland General Hospital
Emergency Medicine Resident

Nadia Juneja, MD
University of Michigan
Emergency Medicine Resident

Jamie "Akiva" Kahn, MD, MBA
Thomas Jefferson University Hospital
Emergency Medicine Resident

Michael M. Khouli, MD
Indiana University
Emergency Medicine/Pediatrics Resident

Brian Kloss, DO, JD, PA-C
SUNY Upstate Medical University
Attending Emergency Physician

Chadd K. Kraus, DO, MPH
EMRA Academic Affairs Representative,
2011-2013
Lehigh Valley Health Network
Emergency Medicine Resident

Michelle Lin, MD, MPH
NYU/Bellevue Hospital Center
Emergency Medicine Resident

Brandon Maughan, MD, MHS
Brown University
Emergency Medicine Chief Resident

K Kay Moody, DO, MPH
Albert Einstein Medical Center
Emergency Medicine Resident

Katherine Nacca, MD
Upstate Medical University
Emergency Medicine Resident

Marisa Oishi, MD, MPH
The Brooklyn Hospital Center
Attending Emergency Physician

Robert Redwood, MD
University of Wisconsin
Emergency Medicine Resident

Ashley Ryles, MD
York Hospital
Emergency Medicine Resident

Sarah M. Schlein, MD
University of Utah
Emergency Medicine Resident

Erin E. Schneider, MD
Former EMRA Health Policy Committee Chair
(2010-2012)
Attending Emergency Physician

Chet Schrader, MD
Baylor Hospital – Garland
Attending Emergency Physician
and Medical Director

Harbir Singh, MD
UT Southwestern Medical Center
Emergency Medicine Resident

Donald E. Stader III, MD
EMRA Immediate Past-President,
2012-2013
Carolinas Medical Center
Emergency Medicine Resident

Joshua Stanton, MD
University of Virginia
Emergency Medicine Resident

Daniel Stein, MD, MPH
Former EMRA Medical Student
Governing Council Chair
(2011-2012)
Oregon Health Sciences University
Emergency Medicine Resident

Seth Trueger, MD
George Washington University
Emergency Medicine Physician and
Health Policy Fellow

Ellie Ventura, MD, MPH
Naval Hospital, Camp Lejeune
Attending Emergency Physician

EMRA Staff Editor
Rachel Donihoo
Emergency Medicine Residents' Association

2012-2013 EMRA Board of Directors

EMRA Staff

Introduction

What is *advocacy*? Simply put, it is a core competency for each of us at the front lines of medicine. Some dismiss advocacy as "just politics," but it is so much more. Advocacy is defined as speaking for a cause, often for a vulnerable person; this is at the very heart of what emergency medicine does, day in and day out.

It is important to remember that you have the *right* to petition the government, which is protected by the First Amendment, to ensure you and your colleagues are receiving equitable treatment under the law. You also have the *responsibility* to advocate for the interests of your patients, who are unable to represent themselves in the American political process.

Each of us can recount an individual experience with a sick patient. Recall that elderly "continuity" septic patient, boarding in your emergency department for 48 hours, handed over time and again, intubated and in critical condition, but without a bed in the ICU. Remember the patient who sat in pain in the hallway, praying for relief, with no call button in sight. We can all bemoan the problem, but how many physicians recognize it as a symptom of the larger issues of overcrowding, boarding, and the need for systemic change?

This handbook was designed to provide you with an introduction to the challenges that face emergency medicine today, and what may be in store in the future. While many will hear about these issues in the news media, little is available for rapid consumption from the emergency physicians' perspective. This handbook, in concert with presentation materials and other educational tools available through EMRA, offers a backbone of knowledge in the increasingly complex administrative, political, and bureaucratic world that surrounds the care of our patients.

Each chapter within this handbook covers an important topic. From a basic outline of the issues, to in-depth resources, to tips on getting involved, each section includes valuable information. If advocacy is a passion of yours, you will have no trouble reading the text from cover to cover. If it is something you find less than interesting, treat the material like you would any other subject; read one chapter each night, or when the book crosses your path.

While it is useful to understand the topics, it also is important to know how to get involved. Participation in the process of improving patient care can take many forms, from local to national; we have provided resources to help you pursue your interests. We also encourage you to seek out information from the EMRA and ACEP websites, which can be great points of reference. Never hesitate to contact EMRA's legislative advisor or Health Policy Committee chair, when the passion strikes you; they are always willing to discuss new and important topics.

We train residents to be good doctors by teaching them what matters. Few, though, have ever heard a lecture on advocacy. Resident education must teach young physicians the skills necessary to advocate for new laws, educate the public on issues that impact health care, and improve the system in which they will work for decades to come.

We are the future of emergency medicine. If we do not speak up for our patients, our colleagues, and ourselves, we will have no room to complain if our ability to provide the right care at the right time in the right place continues to deteriorate. We challenge you to speak up and be heard!

Preface to the Third Edition

How four years can change your perspective. In 2009 I was an emergency medicine resident who believed that advocacy was a critical, but underserved, part of resident education. At that time, a group of young residents undertook the task of writing the first edition of EMRA's *Emergency Medicine Advocacy Handbook* – a resource designed to help their colleagues understand the implications of policy and politics on their future practices. With the passage of the *Patient Protection and Affordable Care Act* (ACA) in March 2010, major revisions to the modern health insurance and delivery system were put in motion, which necessitated the second edition of the handbook.

This year, I was appointed to the Washington State Senate to serve in the state legislature as the Senator for the 26th Legislative District, a privilege that has forever changed my perspective on the issue of advocacy. As an elected official, I sit on the other side of the table and regularly see advocates in 15-minute intervals; I have come to rely on those in other fields to educate me about the environment, education, public safety, and more. While I have learned about subjects far and wide, my heart remains committed to fixing the broken health care system.

From this new vantage point, I can honestly tell you that the need for knowledgeable physicians willing to advocate for real change is more important than ever. Most legislators know little of the complex system or the care that is delivered; they rely on *you* to be the voice of both the patient and provider. Your expertise will guide their policy decisions; your absence will leave a void of information that can lead to poor decision-making. Without you there to help guide policy, erroneous judgments will be made – just as they were two years ago, when Washington State declared chest pain a non-emergent condition and told patients to stop seeking care. Physicians must stand up and help rebuild the system, or live with the consequences of that failure.

Through this third edition of the *Emergency Medicine Advocacy Handbook*, we hope to equip students, residents, and physicians with an understanding of the issues they will confront in practice. Armed with a solid foundation and prepared to face the complicated regulatory process, we hope each physician will play an active role in shaping health care. The Patient Protection and Affordable Care Act initiated the change three years ago, but this is only the beginning. Real work lies ahead, and we must be prepared to lead the charge.

Nathan R. Schlicher, MD, JD, FACEP

Table of Contents

Chapter 1

TEST YOUR KNOWLEDGE

Alison Haddock, MD and Joshua Stanton, MD

How much do you know about emergency medicine advocacy issues? Take this pretest to see where you stand.

1. **The *Emergency Medical Treatment and Active Labor Act* (EMTALA) was passed in 1986. Under this law, any hospital receiving Medicare reimbursement must:**
   a. Require all staff physicians to treat any patient with whom they have established a doctor-patient relationship on an emergent and urgent basis, as needed.
   b. Provide all patients presenting to the emergency department and its surrounding area with a medical screening exam and stabilizing treatment, regardless of their ability to pay.
   c. Staff all emergency departments with board-certified residency-trained emergency physicians.
   d. Develop a method for diverting patients with low-acuity complaints away from the emergency department for care.

2. **Given the experience of Massachusetts, which passed legislation similar to the *Affordable Care Act* (ACA) in 2006, what is expected to happen to emergency department visits after implementation of the ACA?**
   a. ED visits will *decrease* due to improved access to primary care.
   b. ED visits will *decrease* due to patients' fears that the ACA's cost-cutting measures will leave them with a high cost for accessing emergency services.
   c. ED visits will *increase* because patients will have insurance coverage, but will continue to suffer from lack of access to care.
   d. ED visits will *increase* due to the growing number of EDs and emergency physicians spurred by improved funding.

3. **The single most important factor contributing to emergency department crowding is:**
   a. Inadequate availability of emergency physicians and nurses.
   b. Excess emergency department use by low-acuity patients who perceive the ED as the easiest place to receive non-urgent care.
   c. Increased ED length of stay resulting from slow response times of on-call specialists.
   d. Increased ED length of stay after hospital admission resulting from a lack of bed availability.

4. The *Independent Payment Advisory Board* (IPAB) is:
   a. An elected federal task force created to find ways to replace the failing SGR formula.
   b. A panel proposed by the AMA (with ACEP support) as a fair, physician-driven panel to find ways to control Medicare spending.
   c. An independent group, chaired by Alan Simpson and Erskine Bowles, intended to create ways to balance the budget, including cuts to health care spending.
   d. A presidentially appointed board responsible for offering proposals for Medicare savings in years where spending is expected to exceed projected growth.

5. Which of the following lead to difficulties with the retention of consultants willing to take emergency calls for emergency department patients?
   a. Lack of an established physician-patient relationship and higher acuity means that ED patients present a higher liability risk, and taking an ED call can drive up malpractice premiums for specialists.
   b. Regional trauma centers have grown to accommodate regional needs, and smaller hospitals no longer have an incentive to recruit and retain specialists.
   c. The ED patient population includes large numbers of publicly insured and uninsured patients, leading to relatively low compensation rates for specialists taking call.
   d. A and B
   e. A and C
   f. B and C
   g. A, B and C

6. Which of the following is an accurate description of the currently projected trajectory of the physician workforce shortage?
   a. Due to increasing enrollment in medical schools, the shortage is predicted to resolve within the next 15-20 years.
   b. A shortage of more than 100,000 physicians is anticipated by the year 2025.
   c. Surgical specialties will face the most severe shortages, since surgeons typically retire earlier than their non-surgical counterparts.
   d. The shortage will impact urban and rural areas equally, as significantly higher compensation for care delivered in rural areas makes up for the decreased perceived desirability of working in those areas.

7. Funding for services provided by EMTALA is provided by:
   a. The Medicare Prescription Drug, Improvement, and Modernization Act
   b. The Patient Protection and Affordable Care Act
   c. The Health Insurance Portability and Accountability Act
   d. EMTALA is an unfunded mandate.

8. The *Sustainable Growth Rate* (SGR) is a part of the formula used to determine Medicare physician payment rates. It was created with the intent to:
   a. Control the growth in Medicare expenditures for physician services by linking payment updates to the gross domestic product (GDP).
   b. Empower Congress to determine fair and equitable physician reimbursement.
   c. Align incentives to shift patients and the burden of payment from private insurance to public insurance (Medicare/Medicaid).
   d. Estimate the change in total cost for the average physician to operate a medical practice and provide an annual payment update reflecting that change.

9. *Health services research* is a field that studies "how people get access to health care, how much care costs, and what happens to patients as a result of care." Which of the following is a major obstacle to research design in this field?
   a. The large, nationwide administrative databases used by many researchers in the field are being closed and privatized, so their data is more difficult to access.
   b. There is little interest in the data provided by research from these studies, so funding is scarce.
   c. Studies that could generate prospective, randomized data in the field take many years and are extremely expensive.
   d. Research results cannot be generalized nationwide since health care delivery is so varied from state to state.

10. Patients with which insurance status are most impacted by the practice of balanced billing?
    a. Uninsured patients
    b. Publicly insured patients (Medicare/Medicaid)
    c. In-network insured patients
    d. Out-of-network insured patients

11. Increasing utilization of non-physician providers (including nurse practitioners and physician assistants) in the emergency department has been shown to:
    a. Produce clinical outcomes identical to those provided by physicians alone.
    b. Produce slightly worse clinical outcomes, with higher efficiency, than physicians alone.
    c. Produce better outcomes than physicians alone.
    d. No large or conclusive studies on the impact of non-physician providers in the ED have been performed.

12. **Which of the following is a _true_ statement regarding medical liability in the United States?**
    a. Caps on non-economic damages are constitutionally valid in all states and have been shown to decrease health care costs.
    b. When surveyed, fewer than half of physicians admit to practicing defensive medicine; defensive medicine is thought to be a very minor contributor to U.S. health care costs.
    c. Extending the coverage of the Federal Tort Claims Act to care delivered under EMTALA would decrease liability for emergency physicians and consulting specialists and is currently under consideration by the House of Representatives.
    d. The federal government is funding state programs extensively to develop and evaluate alternatives to the current medical liability system, and has already spent more than $1 million per state in 30 states for this effort.

13. **The most important difference between the _Emergency Medicine Action Fund_ and the _National Emergency Medicine Political Action Committee_ (NEMPAC) is:**
    a. The 9-1-1 Network primarily is funded by groups, while the Action Fund relies on _individual_ donations.
    b. The Action Fund was created to influence regulatory processes (at organizations like CMS), but NEMPAC focuses on legislative advocacy.
    c. The Action Fund primarily operates at the _state_ level, whereas NEMPAC emphasizes _federal_ advocacy.
    d. The Action Fund is a partisan organization that contributes solely to progressive causes; however, NEMPAC donates to both conservative and progressive projects and candidates.

14. **The Washington State Health Care Association attempted to retrospectively deny payment for Medicaid patients who visited the ED with conditions ultimately deemed to be "non-urgent" (based on discharge diagnosis). This policy contradicted:**
    a. The Affordable Care Act
    b. The prudent layperson standard
    c. The Employee Retirement Income Security Act (ERISA)
    d. The Billings algorithm

15. **Which of the following has been found to have the greatest impact on the propagation of health inequities and disparities?**
    a. Provider bias
    b. Social determinants of health
    c. Race
    d. Lack of awareness of the existence of disparities

16. **Medical student debt has been a mounting problem for decades. The average student now graduates with more than $150,000 in debt. The primary cause of this increase is:**
    a. Constant growth in the cost of medical education, coupled with changes in the lending laws that reduce subsidized loans and increase the interest burden by making deferment nearly impossible.
    b. Increased use of private loans to cover education and living costs due to the 2008 financial collapse.
    c. Decreased salaries for resident physicians, making loan repayment during residency increasingly difficult
    d. Increased use of loans with variable rates, which steadily have been increasing faster than inflation.

17. **Which of the following is an organization that, as of 2012, provides new board certification only for emergency medicine residency-trained physicians?**
    a. The American Board of Emergency Medicine (ABEM)
    b. The American Osteopathic Board of Emergency Medicine (AOBEM)
    c. The Board of Certification in Emergency Medicine (BCEM)
    d. A and B
    e. A and C
    f. B and C
    g. A, B and C

18. **What is the *Corporate Practice of Medicine Doctrine*?**
    a. A doctrine prohibiting unlicensed individuals or corporations from employing licensed physicians to prevent a conflict of interest between the physician and the employer.
    b. A popular movement of health care systems toward a corporate hospital employee model for all medical specialties, including emergency medicine.
    c. A doctrine modeling joint control of health care services between lay-individuals, corporations, and physicians.
    d. The underlying principle behind the development of patient-centered medical homes (PCMH) and accountable care organizations (ACOs).

19. **In speaking with your congressman about the challenges facing emergency medicine, which of the following types of information should *not* be shared?**
    a. Your personal address or the address of the emergency department where you work.
    b. An explicit request to support or oppose particular legislation.
    c. A patient story with specific identifiable facts about the patient (i.e., name, career).
    d. Any precise statistical information related to your cause.

20. **What resources does EMRA provide to aid in your advocacy education?**
    a. The *Emergency Medicine Advocacy Handbook*
    b. Advocacy Lecture Series
    c. Resident and first-timer's track at ACEP's Leadership and Advocacy Conference
    d. All of the above

TRUE OR FALSE

1. More than one-third of physicians working in U.S. emergency departments are neither board-certified nor residency-trained in emergency medicine.

2. GME funding has been stable for the past 20 years and is viewed to be such a small part of the budget that it is unlikely to be perceived as a real area of savings, protecting it from current budget discussions.

3. Providers are required to report on all measures applicable to their specialty in the *physician quality reporting system* (PQRS) in order to be eligible for the incentive payment adjustment provided by CMS.

4. EMRA is the second-largest specialty association in emergency medicine.

5. The Joint Commission provides certification for primary stroke centers, trauma centers, and primary PCI centers.

6. Any individual or group of individuals may author a bill, but a senator or representative must introduce the bill to Congress.

7. If you visit a legislator's office and request support for a piece of legislation while describing previous specific monetary contributions to a legislator's campaign, you are guilty of illegal and unethical reciprocity.

8. Current "meaningful use" legislation requires electronic medical records to use "push" technology to increase the application of evidence-based practices in order to qualify for incentive payments.

Answer Key

	20. D	10. D
8. F	19. C	9. C
7. T	18. A	8. A
6. T	17. D	7. D
5. F	16. A	6. B
4. T	15. B	5. E
3. F	14. B	4. D
2. F	13. B	3. D
1. T	12. C	2. C
True or False	11. D	1. B

Chapter 2

CROWDING AND BOARDING

Dennis Hsieh, MD, JD and Marisa L. Oishi, MD, MPH

Emergency department *crowding*, a problem that arises when the number of patients exceeds the treatment space capacity, is a national epidemic.[1] Ask emergency physicians about the challenges they face with ED crowding, and they'll share a vast assortment of experiences; yet ask consulting physicians, hospital administrators, or members of the lay public, and puzzled looks may be all you'll get. Even though most Americans have seen and/or heard of crowding and boarding – overflowing waiting rooms, long wait times, and patients on gurneys in the hallway or tucked into corners, to name just a few examples – there is no one more attuned to the dangers and frustrations of this pervasive problem than those who work in the emergency department.

Patients admitted from the emergency department often have to wait there for an inpatient bed to become available, a practice called *boarding*. The practice of boarding admitted patients, coupled with the increasing volume of ED visits,[2,3] has contributed to crowding. The solutions are complex and cannot be found exclusively in the emergency department; the answers lie, instead, in larger system reforms, such as improving access to primary care, balancing surgery schedules, improving turn-around times, increasing inpatient capacity, and other systems-based solutions.[4] Increasing awareness of the issues at hand, exploring potential solutions, and facing the growing impact of health care reform will aid in confronting these challenges.

"Studies have shown that boarding, as opposed to "inappropriate" ED use for non-urgent conditions or the increasing number of ED visits, is the main driver of emergency department overcrowding."

CAUSES OF CROWDING

Emergency department crowding has been a topic of debate in the mainstream media and academic literature since the 1980s, documented by photos of congested EDs, anecdotal cases,[5] and a *Time* magazine cover story focusing on the adverse outcomes suffered as a result of delays in emergency care.[6] In response, the American College of Emergency Physicians (ACEP) Task Force on Overcrowding convened in 1989, publishing a statement on strategies to deal with the issue. Hospitals invested funds to improve staffing and expand EDs, and the number of emergency medicine residency programs increased by 80% to 120 programs. These efforts, however, did not eliminate the problem; almost two decades later, the Institute of Medicine identified several key issues affecting emergency medicine, including the still-persistent issue of ED crowding.[7]

There are three components to ED crowding: *input* (the number of patients coming to the ED), *capacity/throughput* (how quickly patients are seen and move through the ED), and *output* (the ability to disposition patients from the ED).[8]

Input

Between 1997 and 2009, the annual number of ED visits rose from 94.9 million to 136.1 million,[9,10] — almost double what would be expected if aligned with population growth. Initially, many attributed this disproportionate increase to uninsured and Medicaid patients using the ED for non-urgent conditions.[11] This theory has been debunked, however; studies have shown that "inappropriate" and "non-urgent" ED visits, both among the uninsured and the insured, account for only a minor portion of overall emergency department visits.[12,13]

Instead, the rise in visits has been attributed to growing ED use by older populations;[14] decreased access to primary care appointments for acute care;[15] and an increasing number of uninsured, due in part to the economic downturn.[16] The skyrocketing number of ED visits, therefore, highlights a separate problem: *the lack of appropriate and timely access to care for urgent medical problems requiring immediate attention.*

Interestingly, research suggests that (thanks to innovations in capacity and throughput with the implementation of systems such as "fast track') these lower-acuity patients are not contributing to overall emergency department crowding; they only are associated with a negligible increase in ED length of stay and time to first physician contact for other ED visits.[17] On the other hand, many studies show that access to insurance and primary care leads to improved health outcomes,[18] suggesting that – in the absence of insurance and primary care — patients presenting to the ED may be sicker and more likely to require hospitalization. As a result, improving access to insurance and primary care may decrease ED overcrowding by reducing the number of high-acuity patients who require hospitalization, as discussed below.

Capacity and Throughput

While *ED visits* have increased, there has been a corresponding decline in the number of *emergency departments*. In the last 20 years, the number of emergency departments decreased from 5,108 to 4,564.[19] The ability to increase capacity and throughput comes from various flow innovations, including improvements in triage systems and the development of specific areas where low-acuity patients can be seen quickly and efficiently.

Output

In the United States, overall inpatient bed numbers also have decreased over the past 30 years, going from 1.36 million inpatient beds in 1981 to 941,995 in 2010.[20] At the same time, the occupancy rates of these beds across the nation has decreased from 76.7% in 1975 to 67.8% in 2009.[21] This average, however, does not reflect the relative shortage of beds at hospitals facing the most severe ED overcrowding, as 17.7% of EDs see 43.8% of annual ED visits.[22]

Most experts agree that the shrinking number of beds at hospitals with crowded emergency departments has exacerbated the largest contributing factor of crowding: the boarding of admitted patients.[23,24,25,26,27] Studies have shown that boarding, as opposed to "inappropriate" ED use for non-urgent conditions or the increasing number of ED visits, is the main driver of emergency department overcrowding.[28,29,30]

One study, showed that a 10% absolute increase in hospital occupancy resulted in patients waiting, on average, 5% longer to get from the ED to their inpatient beds.[31] Another study showed that one hospital increased its "functional treatment capacity" by 3,175 patient encounters (or by 10,397 hours) annually when it moved admitted patients to inpatient beds within two hours of admission.[32]

In 2008, the ACEP Boarding Task Force released "Emergency Department Crowding: High Impact Solutions"[33] to help better define the problem of crowding and discuss the consequences and potential solutions. The following is based on highlights of the task force findings.

CONSEQUENCES OF CROWDING[34]

Delays in Patient Care

More than one out of 10 critically ill patients waited for more than one hour to see a physician in the emergency department, even though it is well-documented that early diagnosis and treatment leads to better clinical outcomes for the seriously ill.[35] When boarding hours reach above 8.5% of all available emergency department bed hours, there is a significant increase in patients leaving the waiting room before being seen by a physician.[36] The patients who leave are not all low-acuity patients; a number of these walkouts subsequently will require admission when they return.[37] Delays due to boarding may place patients at risk of adverse outcomes and increase medical liability risks for providers.

Increased Complications in Patient Care

There is significant concern for actual patient harm from boarding. Patients with acute coronary syndromes who experience a delay in care may face a significant increase in death, cardiac arrest, heart failure, arrhythmia, and hypotension during times of crowding.[38,39] Increases in medical errors are associated with boarding, such as missing a dose of home medication or a missed ED treatment; these are errors of omission (not commission), precipitated by the simultaneous care of inpatients and new emergency patients.[40,41]

Increased Hospital Lengths of Stay

Total hospital length of stay (LOS) is at least a full day longer among patients boarded in the emergency department, compared to patents with similar illnesses who were promptly placed in inpatient units.[42,43,44] One recent study showed that LOS increased from 5.6 days for those boarding for less than two hours to 8.7 days for those boarding 24 hours or more.[45]

Increased Patient Mortality

Mortality rates among patients spikes during times of crowding; patients who board 12 or more hours may have be at much greater risk than those who board less than two hours.[46,47,48] Research also shows that ICU patients who suffer a delayed transfer to the intensive care unit by more than six hours have a higher mortality rate and increased length of stay compared to those who were transferred promptly.[48] Furthermore, increased boarding has been shown to lead to increased ICU admissions.[49]

Ambulance Diversion

Up to 50% of emergency departments have reported ambulance diversion,[50] the redirecting of incoming ambulances to neighboring hospitals because of a critical lack of ED or inpatient capacity. There is little evidence that diversion actually works to alleviate ED crowding; it is, however, associated with a further delay in patient care, which has been associated with increased mortality.[10]

Financial Losses to Hospital and Physician

The financial impact of emergency care is complicated by payer mix, acuity, and other variables. Medical negligence claims rise during times of crowding; the frequency of medical liability lawsuits increases by a factor of five, simply based on whether a patient waits for more than 30 minutes to be seen by a physician.[51] A 2007 single-center study of historical data found a significantly decreased functional capacity of the ED due to boarders; if patients had been transferred within two hours, the ED beds that were occupied by boarders may have potentially generated $3 million in additional net revenue for the hospital.[52]

While there is some evidence that ED admissions generate more revenue for the hospital than elective admissions,[53,54] other studies suggest the opposite is true. Some research has found that boarding actually *saves* the hospital system money, due to better reimbursement for elective admissions compared with ED admissions,[55] wherein boarding is used as a management practice to maximize overall profits.[56] For example, one analysis showed that each admission from the ED cost the hospital $700.[57] While the financial data is conflicting, these statistics are unable to take into account litigation-related costs, patient satisfaction effects on future patient visits, and other non-monetary factors adversely impacted by the boarding process.

SOLUTIONS: IMPROVING PATIENT ACCESS AND EMERGENCY DEPARTMENT FLOW

Much discussion has occurred in recent years about how to alleviate emergency department overcrowding and boarding. Solutions again focus on the three different components: *input*; *throughput* and *capacity*; and *output*. Many of these solutions, especially those around boarding (output), require a clear commitment by hospital leadership,[58,59,60] as they are hospital-wide or health systems problems and not simply internal emergency department improvements.

The ACEP Boarding Task Force document highlighted not only emergency department solutions (throughput and capacity), but also focused on creating a hospital-wide commitment to improving ED overcrowding by improving efficiencies in inpatient services (output). These concepts have become incorporated into *LEAN, Six Sigma, 5S,* and other process-improvement programs, which are discussed in further detail in the ACEP Boarding Task Force document. On the other hand, strategies around decreasing the number of ED visits (input) are broader systems issues that must take into account the source of patients, payer and acuity mixes, and other local factors. These are discussed briefly below:

Input Solutions (Health Systemwide)
Solution 1: Connecting patients with health care coverage and primary care
• Screen patients for health care coverage.
• Ensure patients without health care coverage apply for insurance coverage.[61]
• Connect patients who are covered and insured with primary care doctors.[62]

Solution 2: Addressing the social and economic determinants of health
• Screen patients for social and economic problems that affect their health.[63]
• Work with hospital staff, hospital administration, community groups, and local government to address the social and economic determinants of health.[64]

LOOKING FORWARD: HEALTH REFORM'S EFFECT ON CROWDING AND BOARDING

The Patient Protection and Affordable Care Act (ACA) of 2010 will increase insurance coverage to include an additional 32 million people within the next 10 years.[65] While some assert that the increase in insurance coverage also will increase primary and preventive care; decrease the number of patient visits to the ED; and ultimately, reduce admissions through the emergency department, our current health care system is poorly prepared to handle the growing volume of insured patients seeking primary care.

The Association of American Medical Colleges Center for Workforce Studies estimates a shortage of 63,000 physicians nationwide by 2015, the year after health care reform is scheduled to take effect.[66] It remains unclear whether the ACA will adequately improve the delivery of care and increase access to primary care and specialist providers – particularly during evening and weekend hours, when 67% of people currently receive acute care services.[67] On the other hand, the ACA encourages the development of new health care delivery models to improve care coordination and increase cost savings and efficiency. Models such as *accountable care organizations* and *patient-centered medical home*s could potentially decrease ED visits and hospital admissions and positively impact crowding by decreasing inpatient boarding.

Although it is unknown what effect the ACA will have on emergency departments, which traditionally have been seen as America's "safety net," some lessons may be learned from the 2006 Massachusetts health care reform. In 2006, Massachusetts passed legislation that moved the state to near-universal coverage. An initial study found that 92% of working adults had a "regular" source of care for when they were sick. Emergency departments, however, continued to see a high volume of visits, a number that has not decreased since legislative implementation.[68] This study also found that adult ED users tended to be sicker, more disabled, more chronically ill, and reported more unmet needs and difficulties obtaining care than other adults in the state.

More recent studies, however, show that over time – as previously uninsured patients become integrated into the health care system – ED usage in Massachusetts may decrease. In the fall of 2010, ED visits dropped for the first time among adults aged 19-64.[69] New research points to an overall 5-8% decrease in ED visits, a decline attributed to a reduction in non-urgent visits for conditions that could be treated in alternate settings; reductions were most pronounced during regular business hours, when physicians' offices are likely to be open.[70] This provides hope that the ACA may improve emergency department crowding in the long term, despite an immediate spike in visits.

NEW GUIDELINES FOR CMS REIMBURSEMENT

As part of health care reform, the Center for Medicare & Medicaid Services (CMS) has propagated new guidelines about ED crowding and boarding that are linked to reimbursement. Some of these measures already are in effect, including: median time from ED arrival to ED departure for discharged patients (OP-18) and patient left before being seen (OP-22).[71] Two others, median time from ED arrival to ED departure (ED-1) and median time from admit decision to ED departure for admitted patients (ED-2), will take effect in 2014. These measures may help incentive hospital-based system changes to decrease ED crowding and boarding.

CONCLUSION

Emergency department crowding – primarily caused by boarding patients admitted to the hospital who do not have timely access to inpatient beds – is not just an emergency medicine problem; it is a hospital-wide problem that needs to be approached by the health care system as a whole. Emergency physicians must advocate at the hospital, local, state, and national levels for system-wide plans to help reduce ED crowding and increase funding and resources that enhance acute care visits without compromising the quality of patient care. ✶

Additional Resources

- *ACEP Practice Resources on ED Crowding:* http://www.acep.org/practres.aspx?id=32050
- *Urgent Matters Toolkit,* SUNY Stony Brook Emergency Department Full Capacity Protocol. Robert Wood Johnson Foundation, 2006: http://www.rwjf.org/pr/product.jsp?id=56493
- Hospitalovercrowding.com website by Peter Viccellio, MD, of SUNY Stony Brook, sponsored by the Emergency Medicine Foundation: http://hospitalovercrowding.com
- Henry J. Kaiser Family Foundation Health Reform Source, http://healthreform.kff.org
- Association of American Medical Colleges Health Care Reform and Physician Workforce Resources: http://aamc.org

Chapter 3

THE IMPACT OF EMTALA

Ramnik S. Dhaliwal, MD, JD

The Emergency Medical Treatment and Active Labor Act (EMTALA) has been described as the largest unfunded federal mandate in health care. Originally designed to protect patients from inappropriate transfers and "dumping," the program has grown to be the basis of the safety net of the American health care system. It is estimated that current costs related to EMTALA have burgeoned to $4.4 billion annually.[1]

THE LAW

In 1986, EMTALA went into effect as part of the Consolidated Omnibus Reconciliation Act (COBRA) of 1985.[2] It established two main obligations on the part of all hospitals that receive any Medicare funding and which maintain an emergency department:[3]

1. For any person who comes to a hospital emergency department, "the hospital must provide for an appropriate medical screening examination...to determine whether or not an emergency medical condition exists," *and*
2. If the screening examination reveals an emergency medical condition, the hospital must "stabilize the medical condition" before transferring or discharging the patient.

Emergency physicians are proud to serve the public 24 hours a day, seven days a week, regardless of an individual's insurance coverage or ability to pay; we serve as the national health care safety net and embrace public trust in treating all who come our way.

Under EMTALA, both of the above must be done, regardless of a patient's insurance coverage or ability to pay.[4] EMTALA compliance is regulated by the Centers for Medicare and Medicaid, a division of the U.S. Department of Health and Human Services (HHS). Touted as a necessary consumer protection law, EMTALA initially was embraced by the public. Unfortunately, EMTALA had no underlying mechanism to secure funding, leaving emergency care providers and hospitals responsible for shouldering the costs of care provided under the mandate.

MEDICAL SCREENING EXAMINATIONS

Any person who arrives at an emergency department and requests examination or treatment for a medical condition *must* be provided a *medical screening examination* (MSE) to determine if an underlying emergency condition exists.

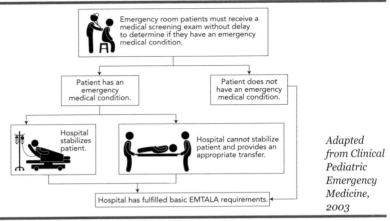

Adapted from Clinical Pediatric Emergency Medicine, 2003

Current provisions allow hospitals to designate members of their health care team to perform the MSE;[5] this must be outlined by the hospital's board of directors. Generally, the MSE is performed by a physician, a nurse, or a midlevel provider. The triage process alone does *not* meet the requirement of the MSE.[6] To satisfy this provision, the examination must be of sufficient detail to uncover an underlying emergency medical condition after a good faith effort. There is no outline specifying what this examination must entail, affording flexibility to the examiner who encounters the spectrum of chief complaints.

Due to the financial pressures many hospitals are experiencing, there has been increasing movement to perform a MSE and then delay further treatment of non-emergent conditions until payment is received. Most notably, the Hospital Corporation of America (HCA) attempted this sort of program.[7] A decision to not continue treatment based on a financial barrier, however, could be perceived as an EMTALA violation. In addition, once a provider has engaged the patient by performing a medical screening exam, he or she has established a relationship with that patient and is obligated by standards of medical liability to provide appropriate care, limiting the ability to withhold care for non-emergent conditions.

THE STABILIZATION REQUIREMENT

Like the screening requirement, the *stabilization requirement* applies to all Medicare-participating hospitals with dedicated emergency departments. The stabilization requirement is triggered when a hospital discovers that an individual has an emergency medical condition. *Screening and stabilizing may not be delayed due to a patient's insurance coverage or ability to pay.* For the stabilization requirement to apply, identification of an emergency medical condition is required.[8] Therefore, if a hospital fails to accurately detect an individual's emergency condition and discharges that patient without stabilizing the medical condition, the hospital may not have violated EMTALA's stabilization provisions. The hospital still may be civilly liable to the individual, however, based upon state medical malpractice claims, if the failure to detect an emergency condition was due to negligence during the screening exam.[9] The definition of an *emergency medical condition* by statute is:[10]

"a medical condition manifesting itself by acute symptoms of sufficient severity (including severe pain) such that the absence of immediate medical attention could reasonably be expected to result in placing the individual's health (or the health of an unborn child) in serious jeopardy, serious impairment to bodily functions, or serious dysfunction of bodily organs; or with respect to a pregnant women who is having contractions that there is inadequate time to effect a safe transfer to another hospital before delivery, or that transfer may pose a threat to the health or safety of the woman or the unborn child."

Federal regulations define an individual as stabilized when there is a reasonable assurance that no material deterioration would result from that individual's transfer or discharge from the hospital or, in the case of women in labor, after delivery of the child and placenta.[11] The physician and the hospital have no EMTALA obligations once a patient has been stabilized, and the patient may be discharged or transferred accordingly as appropriate for the medical condition.[12] The requirement for stabilization is not met with the mere *provision* of triage, unless performed by a member of the medical staff. The screen also must be performed in good faith and without fraudulent intent.

When an emergency medical condition is detected, a hospital may decide to admit the individual for further treatment, sometimes with need for further stabilization as an inpatient. It has been disputed whether the stabilization requirement continues to apply to patients *after* they have been admitted. The Fourth, Ninth, and Eleventh Circuit Courts have held that a hospital has no stabilization duties that are enforceable under EMTALA once an individual has been admitted. More recently, however, the U.S. Court of Appeals for the Sixth Circuit held that the mere admission of an individual, without further treatment, fails to satisfy EMTALA.[13] The defendant hospital petitioned the Supreme Court for review, but the Court declined to hear the case. This case may be irrelevant, however; in February 2012, the U.S. Department of Health and Human Services reiterated its interpretation of EMTALA, ruling that it does not apply to the inpatient setting, even if a patient remains unstable upon admission.[14]

APPROPRIATE TRANSFERS

EMTALA requires a hospital to provide an "appropriate" transfer to another medical facility if a higher level of care or specialized treatment is necessary to stabilize a patient. The receiving hospital must accept such a transfer when it can provide these services, regardless of a patient's insurance or fiscal status. In addition, a patient may be transferred only if a physician certifies that the medical benefits expected from the transfer outweigh the risks, or if a patient makes a request in writing after being informed of the risks and benefits associated with the transfer. In either case, all of the following also must apply:[15]

1. The patient has been treated and stabilized as far as possible within the capabilities of the transferring hospital.
2. The transferring hospital must continue providing care en-route with the appropriate personnel and medical equipment to minimize risk.
3. The receiving hospital has been contacted and agrees to accept the transfer.

4. The receiving hospital has the facilities, personnel and equipment to provide necessary treatment.
5. Copies of the medical records accompany the patient.

According to statute, a patient is considered stable if the treating physician determines that he or she will have no material deterioration during transfer between facilities. Unanticipated adverse outcomes or deterioration do not typically constitute an EMTALA violation.[16] Given the severity of the penalties involved, most hospitals include EMTALA language in transfer forms to avoid the possibility that a retrospective review of a case might be interpreted as a violation.

PHYSICAL AREA OF COVERAGE

Regulatory revisions to EMTALA in 2003 by HHS also have broadened its applicability from patients arriving at an emergency department to patients arriving on a "hospital campus."[17] This is defined as the physical area up to 250 yards from the main hospital building, including parking lots, driveways, sidewalks, administrative entrances, and areas that may bypass the emergency department, such as labor and delivery. Walk-in clinics, urgent care facilities, and outpatient treatment areas located at satellite facilities that do not provide emergency services do *not* fall under the umbrella of EMTALA law.[18]

THE PENALTIES

The Office of Inspector General for the Department of Health and Human Services and the Centers for Medicare & Medicaid Services (CMS) are responsible for investigating complaints of EMTALA violations. An EMTALA violation may result in fines to the individual physician and the hospital, each up to $50,000 per incident, plus termination of their Medicare and Medicaid contracts.

Currently, there is a two-year statute of limitations for civil enforcement of any violation. Citation for a CMS violation does not require any legal conviction or adverse outcome, and is not typically covered by standard malpractice insurance plans. Receiving facilities may sue to recover damages and fiscal losses suffered as a result of an inappropriate transfer from another hospital in violation of EMTALA. If receiving hospitals fail to report EMTALA violations, they may be subject to misdemeanor charges. If a patient refuses examination or treatment in the absence of coercion, there is no EMTALA violation. On-call physician specialists who fail to come to the emergency department after having been called by an emergency physician also may be found in violation of EMTALA;[19] hospitals can be found liable when their providers or policies cause EMTALA violations.

THE PROBLEM

Although, in spirit, EMTALA was intended to support the rights of the individual indigent patient, the unanticipated consequences of the law have resulted in decreased access to care for many. A 2003 Government Accountability Office (GAO) report showed the specific effects of medical liability premiums on emergency and trauma specialists. The GAO study documented that in medical liability crisis states, access to emergency care was *reduced* (particularly for trauma and obstetrical services); delays in care were more frequent; transfers of patients increased; and the availability of on-call specialists to emergency departments was reduced, due to the combined burdens of EMTALA and a challenging liability climate.[20] Further, the large quantity of uncompensated care provided by emergency physicians and hospitals every day put a large financial burden on these already strained resources.

Since EMTALA was signed into law, EDs have experienced a dramatically increasing volume of patients. From 1997 to 2000, ED use increased by 14% to 108 million visits annually; by 2009, the number of ED visits reached 136.1 million.[21] Researchers speculate that EMTALA has been responsible for part of this increase in volume, requiring many EDs to operate at or above their capacities.[22, 23,24]

Uncompensated care delivered by nonfederal community hospitals grew from $6.1 billion in 1983 to $39.1 billion in 2009.[25,26] Furthermore, 55% of emergency care goes uncompensated;[27] and emergency physicians currently provide more uncompensated care than any other physician specialty, according to CMS. A 2003 American Medical Association (AMA) report revealed that each emergency physician in 2000 averaged $138,399 in EMTALA-related lost revenue per year, with over one-third providing more than 30 hours of EMTALA-related charity care each week. By stark contrast, physicians in other specialties averaged less than six hours of EMTALA-related care each week, and they incurred only about $12,300 in EMTALA-related lost revenue per year.[28]

The effects of unfunded care have been widespread, contributing to much of the strain affecting the current U.S. medical system. As outlined in other chapters, hundreds of hospitals and emergency departments have closed, waiting times have increased, overcrowding and boarding have reached a critical point, on-call physician coverage has broken down, and many hospitals currently function near or at their surge capacities. It is doubtful that federal funding will be provided in the current economic climate to make the requirements of EMTALA less onerous. Indirect funding through additional Medicare payments for physicians who perform emergency-related services has been considered, but is unlikely. If additional funding is provided, this likely would result in a corresponding decrease in reimbursement in other areas.

EXPANDING PATIENT POPULATION AND BURDEN

According to the Congressional Budget Office (CBO), the Affordable Care Act would reduce the number of uninsured by about 32 million, leaving about 23 million nonelderly residents uninsured.[29] Researchers project that of those remaining uninsured, 26% will be illegal immigrants; 38% will be patients eligible for Medicaid or Children's Health Insurance Program (CHIP), but unenrolled; 8% will qualify for an affordability exemption from the individual mandate penalties; and 28% will be those opting to pay penalties rather than obtain health insurance, as required under the individual mandate.[30]

Some experts believe these changes in coverage will result in more emergency department visits and longer waits, as insured patients strain the capacity of the primary care system and are less reluctant to present to the ED for care once they have insurance. In Massachusetts, the results of state-based health care reform are still difficult to interpret. Since 2006, when the state mandated that its citizens carry health insurance, visits to emergency departments have remained relatively stable. Despite the mandate, ED visit rates mirror those of neighboring states New Hampshire and Vermont – an ambiguous finding that begs further investigation.[31]

Emergency physicians may benefit from securing some compensation from the 32 million newly insured Americans who otherwise would have been received uncompensated care under EMTALA. Since the new legislation does not directly address EMTALA-related care, however, emergency physicians will continue to provide uncompensated care to the 23 million Americans who remain uninsured. Furthermore, to pay for the Medicaid expansion, the federal government plans to cut funding to safety net hospitals previously earmarked for care of these uninsured.[31]

LIABILITY REFORM

Many organizations have proposed that liability reform and protections for EMTALA-related care under the Federal Tort Claims Act would provide an alternative compensation model with minimal costs. At the federal level, the American College of Emergency Physicians (ACEP) helped introduce legislation in 2011 in the form of H.R. 157, "The Health Care Safety Net Enhancement Act of 2011." In its current form, this would extend liability coverage to emergency physicians under the Public Health Safety Act, which would insure them as federal employees with "sovereign immunity."[32] While this legislation gained traction in the U.S. House of Representatives and was included as part of a larger liability reform bill, the legislation has not moved through the Senate. The bill was reintroduced in the 113th Congress in January 2013. At time of press, it has bipartisan support from 30 cosponsors in the House.

CONCLUSION

The purpose of EMTALA is to ensure equal treatment for any person seeking emergency care. Emergency physicians are proud to serve the public 24 hours a day, seven days a week, regardless of an individual's insurance coverage or ability to pay; we serve as the national health care safety net and embrace public trust in treating all who come our way. Nevertheless, EMTALA has shifted public policy responsibilities onto hospitals and physicians. It does not require health insurance companies, the federal government, nor individuals to pay for any mandated services. Emergency physicians and their on-call colleagues are beginning to demand a mechanism to secure funding and/or limit liability for the providers of EMTALA-mandated services. State-level attempts to retroactively deem care provided under the EMTALA mandate to have been non-emergent, thus not meriting reimbursement (under Medicaid or other state health plans) to the providers of care, will exacerbate the strain associated with EMTALA. Failure to protect the safety net will result in further deterioration of a system already in crisis. ✱

With thanks to H. Samuel Ko, MD, MBA and Edwin Lopez, MD for their authorship of a previous version of this chapter.

Chapter 4

"NON-EMERGENT" VISITS AND THE PRUDENT LAYPERSON STANDARD

Jordan Celeste, MD

In the lay press, in discussions with physicians from other specialties, and – most alarmingly – in conversations with our legislators, we often hear that patients in the emergency department "don't need to be there." When these dangerous words begin to take the form of actual policy, it is our responsibility as emergency physicians to advocate for our patients' right to emergency care. In order to refute the fallacies, it is important to understand the actual data on "non-emergent" visits to the ED.

"NON-EMERGENT" VISITS TO THE EMERGENCY DEPARTMENT

Limiting visits to the emergency department has been proposed as a cost-saving measure for the U.S. health care system for many years. Research suggests, however, that the high cost of medicine cannot be attributed to emergency department utilization. While EDs are seeing more than 136 million visits a year,[1] emergency care comprises fewer than 2% of our country's health care expenditures.[2]

> *"The prudent layperson standard turns logical patient protection into law; veering from this standard sends the dangerous message that patients are expected to diagnose themselves."*

The argument that most patients do not need to be in the emergency department is often built on decades-old data[3] or on the misinterpretation of studies designed for another purpose (such as the Billings study, discussed later in this chapter). The Centers for Disease Control and Prevention (CDC) reports that only a very small portion – less than 8% – of emergency department visits are for conditions deemed "non-urgent."[4] Moreover, the CDC defines "non-urgent" conditions as those which require care within 2-24 hours; at no point are these visits stated to be "inappropriate" or "unnecessary."[5]

Telling patients that they don't belong in the emergency department violates one of the founding tenets of the specialty – that *a patient's symptoms define the emergency.*[6] Patients present to the ED with symptoms, not final diagnoses. A patient comes to the emergency department with chest pain because he is worried he's having a heart attack; the fact that he ultimately may be diagnosed with gastroesophageal reflux should not discourage him from seeking medical care. Likewise, patients with life-threatening diseases should not be forced to avoid care because of financial concerns.

THE PRUDENT LAYPERSON STANDARD

The *prudent layperson standard* grew out of the insurance environment of the early 1980s. In 1986 the U.S. Congress passed EMTALA, setting the standard that hospitals must provide care to anyone needing emergency treatment. Private insurers, however, routinely would require prior authorization for emergency department visits or deny payments for visits that they deemed inappropriate for that care setting, often based on a retrospective review or discharge diagnosis. If an individual wanted insurance to cover an emergency treatment, the patient was expected to contact his or her insurer for approval *prior* to the ED visit. If an individual sought care in the emergency department and his or her insurer later deemed that the final diagnosis did not require emergency care, the insurer would refuse to pay for the visit.[7]

In response to such potentially dangerous and unfair requirements, many states enacted *prudent layperson standards*. Maryland, in 1993, was the first to do so; 47 states ultimately passed legislation that supported a patient's right to seek care in the emergency department.[8] The Balanced Budget Act of 1997 extended prudent layperson standards to Medicare and Medicaid managed care plans. The language from the act eloquently states what, at its core, is a simple concept:

"The term 'emergency medical condition' means a medical condition manifesting itself by acute symptoms of sufficient severity (including severe pain) such that a prudent layperson, who possesses an average knowledge of health and medicine, could reasonably expect the absence of immediate medical attention to result in:

(i) placing the health of the individual (or, with respect to a pregnant woman, the health of the woman or her unborn child) in serious jeopardy,

(ii) serious impairment to bodily functions, or

(iii) serious dysfunction of any bodily organ or part."[9]

Although nearly every state had passed legislation establishing its own prudent layperson standards, there was also intense interest in enacting *federal* legislation; self-insured health plans were still exempt from the state mandates via the federal Employee Retirement Income Security Act (ERISA).[7] The American College of Emergency Physicians (ACEP) was very active in advocating for a federal prudent layperson standard, supporting legislation, and recruiting other organizations to follow its lead. Senator Benjamin Cardin (D–Maryland) included prudent layperson language in an amendment, known as the Patient's Bill of Rights, which was included as part of the Patient Protection and Affordable Care Act in 2010.[10] After 15 years of advocacy, ACEP finally saw its efforts realized with the passage of the ACA.

STATE EFFORTS TO LIMIT VISITS

Efforts to limit emergency department visits drew national attention after the Washington State Health Care Authority (HCA) began exploring ways to trim the state Medicaid budget. The movement began in mid-2011 with a list of 700 "non-urgent" conditions, and limited Medicaid enrollees to three emergency department visits a year for any of these conditions. This list was based on a patient's ultimate diagnosis after an ED visit, not his or her chief complaint. Working with other stakeholder organizations, the Washington State Chapter of ACEP quickly responded.

After months of regulatory meetings followed by legal action, the emergency physicians and their allies were able to halt implementation in the courts. After a brief attempt by the HCA to use retrospective denial to block payment for even a single emergency department visit it deemed non-urgent, Washington ACEP proposed alternative cost-saving measures that could be used in the state and ultimately were passed by the state legislature.[11]

While Washington served as a proving ground for legislation seeking to restrict emergency department visits, other states – including Tennessee, Kentucky, and New Hampshire – have explored similar strategies. With increasing budgetary difficulties, the trend of limiting emergency department visits based on lists of "non-urgent" or "non-emergent" diagnoses is likely to continue.

INCORRECT TOOL, INACCURATE METHOD

In an effort to evaluate primary care delivery systems, Professor John Billings, director of the NYU Wagner Health Policy and Management Program, developed an algorithm that examined emergency departments. His original paper, published in 2000, stated: "The algorithm is not intended as a triage tool or a mechanism to determine whether ED use is appropriate for required reimbursement by a managed care plan...Nor was it intended to assess appropriateness of ED utilization. Use of the emergency department for minor conditions may well be rational and appropriate if a patient has no other source of care. Moreover, assessment of urgency by patients can be problematic, and labeling ED use for primary care treatable conditions as inappropriate may misallocate responsibility to the patients themselves."[12]

These statements reflect the philosophy behind the prudent layperson standard; the methodology behind the Billings algorithm does not. The algorithm relies on patient diagnosis and not chief complaint, and retrospectively designates emergency department visits as "non-emergent" based on probabilities derived from a small sample of patients in the Bronx.

There also are other methodological issues with the algorithm. It excludes admitted patients, thus selecting for patients with less acute illness, and is unable to assess what motivated patients to seek emergency care in the first place. It cannot evaluate if patients were concerned about a life-threatening condition, or referred to the ED by a primary care doctor, or unable to access care in any location other than the emergency department.

CONCLUSION

Emergency care is not a major driving force behind rising costs in the U.S. health care system; instead, it provides a critical service at a relatively low cost. Emergency departments are a vital component of the system and provide a crucial safety net for millions of Americans. The average person facing a medical emergency should be able to seek care in an emergency department and know that the care will be covered by his or her health plan. The prudent layperson standard turns this logical patient protection into law; veering from this standard sends the dangerous message that patients are expected to diagnose themselves. Emergency physicians need to be vigilant – explaining the risks associated with this incorrect logic, while also highlighting the critical role of emergency medicine in the American health care system. *

Chapter 5

ACCESS TO CARE: SYSTEM-BASED ISSUES

Michelle Lin, MD, MPH

The Emergency Medical Treatment and Labor Act (EMTALA) virtually guarantees the right of every American to access emergency care without regard for an individual's ability to pay.[1] Due to this unique obligation, emergency departments nationwide have become a de facto safety net for those unable to access medical care in other venues. While politicians may continue to equate access to *emergency* care with access to *medical* care, there is tremendous strain on emergency networks to effectively fulfill this high-capacity role.[2]

> Faced with overcrowding, diversion, transport delays, and increasing wait times, our current reality has become increasingly incongruent with the vision of a health care system that is able to deliver timely and appropriate emergency medical care.

The enactment of health care reform under the Patient Protection and Affordable Care Act (ACA) is projected to extend health insurance coverage to 34 million citizens.[3] The legislation contains measures to regulate insurance companies, improve coverage, and advance the quality and efficiency of care delivered, while attempting to decrease skyrocketing costs. As part of the improvement of coverage, the ACA mandates a minimum standard benefits package, which includes coverage for emergency care under the *prudent layperson* standard. The implementation of the national prudent layperson standard will prevent insurance companies from denying payment for visits retrospectively deemed "non-emergent," and allow patients access to timely emergency care without the threat of unmanageable out-of-pocket bills.

Insurance coverage, however, does not guarantee access to care. Emergency department and trauma center closures, overcrowding, lack of on-call specialists, unequal geographic distribution and other disparities have resulted in a broken system. Access to quality emergency care for too many Americans is limited – and in some cases, nonexistent.

RISING DEMAND AND LONGER DELAYS

According to the most recent National Hospital Ambulatory Medical Care Survey (NHAMCS) published by the CDC, there were a total of 136 million emergency visits in 2009, an increase of 9.9% from the previous year.[4] In addition, the proportion of uninsured patients rose from 15.4% to 19.0%, reflective of a corresponding increase in the number of uninsured Americans nationwide (an increase from 46.3 million to 50.7 million). These increases are consistent with a historical trend, which has seen a rise in ED visits of 32% over a ten-year period from 1999 to 2009.

In 2011, with implementation of certain early provisions of the ACA, the number of uninsured Americans decreased for the first time in ten years, from a record high of 48.6 million in 2010 to 46.6 million in 2011.[5] A portion of this gain can be attributed to the extension of coverage for young adults (age 19 to 26), who now may retain coverage under their parents' plans. The creation of a temporary high-risk pool for individuals with pre-existing conditions who were previously denied insurance will continue to provide coverage to some uninsured until health insurance exchanges begin operation in 2014. The remainder of the increase in coverage will take place through extended eligibility for Medicaid.

Starting in 2014, states that choose to participate in the federally funded expansion will be expected to increase their Medicaid income eligibility to 133% of the federal poverty level (to $14,856 for an individual and $30,657 for a family of four). CMS estimates that an additional 34 million Americans will be newly insured by 2019, resulting in a significant increase in demand for health care services, including emergency care.[3] In Massachusetts, where compulsory health insurance has been in place since 2006, ED visits are still rising at rates at or higher than before the law was enacted.[6]

Longer delays for patients awaiting treatment are concurrent with increases in emergency department volumes. Mean wait times increased by 25% from 2003 to 2009 (from 46.5 minutes to 58.1 minutes), with the most significant delays seen in EDs with higher volumes (>50,000 patients annually) and those located in urban settings.[7] Additionally, ambulance diversion was associated with increased wait times, as was ED boarding of admitted patients. Escalating demand continues to strain emergency departments that are already struggling with limited resources and physical space.

HOSPITAL CLOSURES AND A SAFETY NET IN CRISIS

Compounding the problem is a net decline in the number of emergency departments nationwide (a decrease of 27% in the past 19 years, from 2,446 to 1,779).[8] These closures have resulted in increased ambulance diversions and overcrowding at adjacent facilities, and have taxed the capacity of the emergency care network.[9] ED closures primarily have been attributed to economic factors and low profitability, with increasing odds of closure associated with for-profit status; location in a competitive market; and most alarmingly, safety-net status.

While public safety-net hospitals represent only 2% of hospitals in the U.S., they provide almost a quarter of all uncompensated care nationwide.[10] They also treat a substantially higher proportion of publically insured patients than their peer institutions, with reimbursement seldom covering costs. The financial challenges that face safety-net providers are anticipated to deepen with reductions in *disproportionate share hospital* (DSH) payments under the ACA, starting in 2014.[11] These payments are allocated to hospitals that provide an excessive amount of uncompensated care; many safety-net hospitals depend on them for solvency. Over the next five years, DSH funding will be cut in half, a financial loss that is intended to be offset by increasing numbers of insured patients under the new health care law. Many fear these offsets will be insufficient, however, leading to financial difficulties and an increased burden on the already tenuous safety-net system.

INCREASING COMPLEXITY AND AN AGING POPULATION

Not only are patient volumes increasing, the acuity of illness and co-morbid conditions continues to escalate among patients presenting to emergency departments. According to the NHAMCS, non-urgent (triage acuity level 5) visits comprised only 7.7% of total ED visits in 2009.[12] Well over 50% of visits were categorized as emergent or urgent. With an aging population and advancing health care needs and desires, emergency departments continue to face new challenges.

As of 1993, elderly patients accounted for nearly one in five emergency patients; in the subsequent ten-year period from 1993 to 2003, the number of ED patients aged 65 and older increased by 34%.[13,14] In a 1992 survey of emergency physicians, nearly half reported increased difficulty in caring for geriatric patients; the majority also believed that the amount of research and training dedicated to caring for elderly patients with complex disease was inadequate.[15] Elderly patients in emergency departments are significantly more likely to be admitted (2.5 to 4.6 times) and are five times more likely to face admission to the ICU than non-elderly patients.[16]

Older patients also are at higher risk for adverse events related to health care, such as falls and medication errors; and, despite their increased triage acuity in comparison to younger patients, may even be at increased risk for *undertriage*.[17] A number of geriatric-specific EDs have been established in recent years, implementing structural interventions to provide more specialized care for the aging population.[18,19] While geriatric EDs represent a growing trend, few facilities are capable of devoting resources exclusively to care of the elderly.

EMERGENCY MEDICINE WORKFORCE

As critical as physical infrastructure is to the delivery of timely, quality emergency department care, *human* resources – emergency physicians, nurses, and allied health staff – are just as important. In 2008, there were 39,000 emergency physicians in the United States, 69% of whom were either residency-trained or board-certified.[20] To meet the challenges of an aging population and increased utilization, it is estimated that it would take at least another 25 years to fully staff all EDs with board-certified emergency physicians.[21] In the meantime, alternative solutions (such as utilizing midlevel and physician providers who are not board-certified in emergency medicine, as well as new documentation and delivery efficiency strategies) need to be explored.

NURSING SHORTAGES

There are approximately 90,000 nurses working in EDs throughout the U.S.; they provide the bulk of direct patient care.[22] As our country's population ages, the relative shortage of nurses is projected to reach 500,000 full-time positions by 2025. This may impact EDs more than other care areas; the pace, acuity and stress of emergency work can lead to relatively high turnover. Nationwide, approximately 12% of the registered nursing positions for which hospitals are recruiting are for work in EDs, trailing only medical/surgical and critical care units.[23] Additionally, many hospitals have had to reduce previous requirements such as ICU experience or duration from nursing graduation to fill open spots; this trend potentially compounds shortages in staffing.

SPECIALTY CARE

Even patients who are cared for by a well-trained team of emergency providers may not have adequate access to the care they require. While the acuity and complexity of emergency department visits has increased, access to "on-call" specialist physicians has become limited in many facilities.

According to a 2005 survey by the American College of Emergency Physicians (ACEP), nearly three in every four emergency department medical directors reported inadequate specialist coverage in their EDs.[24] The top five specialties cited were orthopedics; plastic surgery; neurosurgery; ear, nose and throat; and hand surgery. To retain specialist coverage, many hospitals (50% in a 2010 American Hospital Association survey) provide stipends to on-call specialists, regardless of whether or not they see patients.[25] Despite this, trends point to a decrease in on-call coverage across many different specialties in all regions of the country.[26]

PEDIATRIC EMERGENCY MEDICINE

The challenge of *access* to quality pediatric emergency care remains a significant system-based problem. Children and adolescents made up roughly 20% of U.S. emergency department visits in 2007; infants less than 12 months of age had the highest per capita ED utilization of any population group.[27] Despite this, only 6% of EDs have all the supplies necessary to handle pediatric emergencies, and only about half have 85% of these supplies.[28] While many urban locales have specialized children's hospitals and emergency departments, the vast majority of children are cared for in general emergency departments. There, lack of resources, missed nuances of pediatric medicine, and reduced specialist coverage can present challenges to the provision of consistent, quality care.

RURAL EMERGENCY MEDICINE

Access to adequate emergency care for the 60 million Americans who live in rural areas also is problematic. Though 21% of the U.S. population lives in rural locales, only 12% of emergency physicians (including non-residency-trained emergency physicians) practice in these settings.[29] Access to specialty care in rural EDs is limited, as well; rural EDs provide only 44% of the referral and specialist options of those situated in urban centers, with particular deficits in cardiology, neurosurgery, neurology and gastroenterology.[30] Additional studies suggest that trauma mortality, especially for pediatric and geriatric patients, is significantly higher in rural areas.[31] Forty-seven million Americans currently live outside the so-called "golden hour" (more than 60 minutes from a Level I or Level II trauma center); of these, most reside in rural America.[32]

CONCLUSION

Although each person in America is legally guaranteed the right to receive emergency care, regardless of insurance or immigration status, the nature and quality of this care varies greatly. Faced with overcrowding, diversion, transport delays, and increasing wait times, our current reality has become increasingly incongruent with the vision of a health care system that is able to deliver timely and appropriate emergency medical care. Rising volumes, hospital closures, workforce shortages, and unequal geographic distribution create an increasing bottleneck that promises only to worsen.

The greatest disparities in access persist for pediatric patients and those who live in rural areas. With the implementation of national health care reform under the ACA, emergency utilization is projected to increase as more Americans become newly insured. The imperative to improve access to outpatient and primary care visits and reduce overcrowding will become even more pressing in the near future. Together, as emergency physicians, we must continue to advocate for our patients and preserve the viability of our nation's emergency medical system, so that we may continue to provide timely, appropriate, and quality emergency care for all individuals. ✶

With thanks to Anthony Foianini, MD for his authorship of a previous version of this chapter.

Chapter 6

COVERAGE AND UTILIZATION

William Fleischman, MD

The American health care system is comprised of a patchwork of constantly evolving delivery organizations. Unlike single-payer systems in other countries, care in the United States is covered by a multitude of *payers*. These include employer-purchased private insurance, individually purchased private insurance, Medicare, Medicaid, and other public programs (such as military and veteran affairs organizations). Different laws apply to different types of insurance; access to care, emergency department utilization and reimbursement can vary significantly according to an individual's insurance program.

TYPES OF INSURANCE

Private

The private insurance market functions as a cost-sharing and risk-management pool, where individuals or their employers pay set monthly premiums, while insurers cover much of the beneficiaries' health care costs. There are cost-sharing mechanisms in place aimed at reducing and redirecting care; so beneficiaries may be responsible for the initial portion or a certain percentage of costs (deductibles), as well as per visit/procedure payments (copayments).

In 2010 64% of Americans had some private insurance coverage (including people with dual coverage), while approximately 53% had private insurance alone. The percentage of privately covered individuals has dropped steadily in the past 20 years (Figure 1).[1] Private insurance premiums have surged by 172% since 1999 – more than four times the rate of inflation – significantly increasing health care costs for the majority of Americans.[2]

Employer-Purchased Programs. Most individuals whom the lay public considers "insured" have employer-provided coverage. The expansion of employer-based insurance began during World War II, when wage control laws did not apply to fringe benefits like health insurance.[3] The expansion continued after the war, in large part because these plans allowed businesses to provide a form of tax-free compensation to employees. In 2010, approximately 55% of Americans were covered by insurance purchased by their employers.[1]

Individual Plans. In 2010, only a small proportion of Americans (9.8%) were covered by direct-purchase or individual insurance plans.[1] One of the major reasons for the development of the ACA was the lack of affordable insurance available to individuals. With employers facing escalating health insurance costs, employees were being dropped from group programs, leaving them on their own to find individual health insurance – an option that can be prohibitively expensive. The ACA will create third-party markets through the health insurance exchanges; this is anticipated to increase access to affordable coverage for individuals who do not have coverage through their employers. The Congressional Budget Office (CBO) estimates nine million people will become insured through the exchanges.

Public

Government coverage has been steadily expanding and now covers 31% of all covered individuals (Figures 1,2). Of note, while only 31% are government-insured, government dollars made up nearly *half* of the $2.6 trillion in U.S. health expenditures in 2010.[4] Coverage is provided via a variety of organizations and funds.

Figure 1. Historical Insurance Coverage Trend, 1987-2010

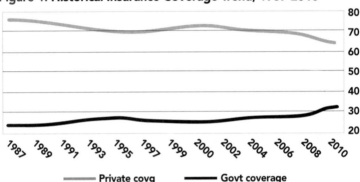

Adapted from the 2010 U.S. Census Population Report.[1] Includes people with dual coverage.

Medicare

In 1965 President Lyndon B. Johnson signed into law the creation of Medicare and Medicaid, profoundly changing the landscape of American medicine. Medicare is the most influential player in our nation's health care. It sets national standards for hospital and physician reimbursement rates, funds the majority of graduate medical education, and is the second largest provider of health insurance nationally (after Medicaid), covering 48.7 million Americans in 2011.[5] Beneficiaries include people 65 and older, the disabled, and people requiring renal dialysis. Prior to 1965, half of older Americans had no health insurance; by 1970, 97% were covered. The number of Medicare beneficiaries increased from 19 million in 1965 to over 48 million in 2011, and is expected to reach 81 million by 2030.[5]

Medicare consists of four separate parts. *Part A* covers hospital inpatient services and skilled nursing care. *Part B* covers outpatient, ED visits and physician services. *Part C* medicare advantage gives beneficiaries the option to have private insurance coverage, which the government pays for in fixed premiums. *Part C* essentially is a managed care program; over 25% of beneficiaries chose that option in 2011.[5] Medicare *Part D* was added in 2006 to cover prescription medications.

Beneficiaries can either enroll in privately run plans to cover prescription drug costs, or enroll in Medicare Advantage plans that include prescription coverage.

Funding for the program comes from mandatory contributions by both employees and employers, premiums and co-payments paid by beneficiaries, and general tax revenues. In 2011 the total Medicare expenditures were $549 billion, with $530 billion in income and $325 billion in reserves.[5]

Once contentious, Medicare quickly became sacred. Beneficiaries, given their power as a voting bloc, have made it politically difficult to alter or reduce Medicare benefits. Expenditures continue to rise rapidly; cost containment programs have, so far, been largely unsuccessful. Proposals to limit spending have focused on reducing payments to hospitals and physicians. The Medicare sustainable growth rate (SGR) conundrum dramatically illustrates this. Rapidly rising health care costs and an aging population will continue to put pressure on the government to limit expenses, but competing political pressures will remain to expand coverage for new medical treatments.

Medicaid

Medicaid was enacted almost as an afterthought to Medicare to provide medical coverage to the poor. Initially intended to supplement existing state entitlement programs, Medicaid has grown into the largest health insurer in the U.S., and is the tool most used by the federal and state governments to expand health care coverage. While *Medicare* largely is a single-payer (the federal government) insurer, *Medicaid* is administered by the individual states and funded from both state and matching federal funds. States must meet national standards to receive federal funds, but each state sets its own regulations. This has created, in essence, 50 different programs.

Medicaid's role is immense, covering more than 55 million beneficiaries in 2011 at a cost of $427 billion.[6] It provided coverage for more than 27 million children, as well as many adult beneficiaries, including eight million disabled Americans.[6] The program also covered nearly 40% of total nursing home costs in the U.S.[6] Notably, the elderly and disabled comprised 25% of Medicaid beneficiaries in 2009, but accounted for 66% of its budget.[6] The program has grown as health care costs have risen faster than inflation and GDP and is expected to expand rapidly when the 2014 ACA reforms are implemented. The Congressional Budget Office (CBO) estimates that ACA reforms will add 11 million beneficiaries to Medicaid and CHIP by 2021.[7]

CHIP – The Children's Health Insurance Program

CHIP was signed into law in 1997 to provide health insurance to children (and in some states, their parents) of families whose incomes are too high to qualify for Medicaid, but who can't afford private coverage. CHIP is administered by the state as either part of its existing Medicaid program or separately; the federal government provides matching funds to states similar to Medicaid. CHIP covered close to eight million children in 2011 at a cost of nearly $12 billion.[8]

Other Programs

About 4.4% of the U.S. population has some type of military health insurance.[9]
Depending on a variety of factors, veterans are eligible for coverage under the
Tricare program and/or the Veteran Affairs Healthcare (VAH) system, which had
a 2012 budget of nearly $51 billion.[10] Also of note, the Indian Health Service serves
about two million American Indians and had a federally subsidized budget of $4.3
billion in 2012.[11]

Figure 2. U.S. Health Care Coverage, 2010

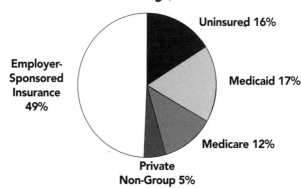

Adapted from the KCMU/Urban Institute analysis of 2011 ASEC Supplement to the CPS.

THE UNINSURED

In 2012, the Census Bureau estimated that 48.6 million Americans (15.7%) were
uninsured, a slight drop from the 16.3% estimate of 2010.[9] The ACA provisions
extending parental coverage to children under age 26 reduced uninsured rates
among young adults by about 6%; this is thought to be the primary reason behind
the drop in uninsured patients between 2010 and 2012.[12]

In general, the last decade has been marked by an incremental increase in the
uninsured population (Figure 3). Most of the uninsured are younger than 45,
with the highest uninsured rates among 19 to 34-year-olds. Approximately 28
million (57%) of the uninsured work part-time or full-time. African-Americans
and Hispanics have the highest uninsured rates; approximately 81% are American
citizens. Southern and Western states have higher rates of uninsured than
Northeast and Midwestern states (18% vs 12%).[9]

The CBO estimates that by 2021 the ACA will reduce the number of uninsured
by 30 million, leaving another estimated 30 million uninsured. The CBO report
was updated after the Supreme Court decision on the ACA, and concludes
that the Court's decision will result in about four million more uninsured by
2021, mainly as a result of some states opting not to implement the expanded
Medicaid coverage.[13] The remaining uninsured will be somewhat older (given the

extension of parental coverage mentioned above), and with incomes too high to meet expanded Medicaid thresholds but too low to afford insurance premiums. Undocumented immigrants also will make up a substantial portion of the uninsured, as they do now, since the ACA reforms do not affect them.[14]

Figure 3. Number Uninsured and Uninsured Rate: 1987 to 2011

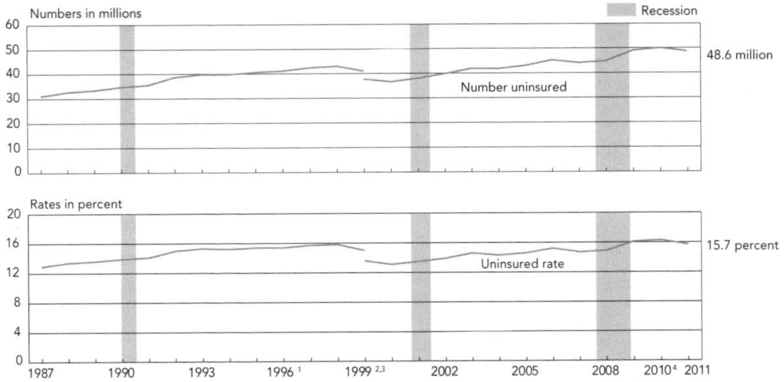

[1]The data for 1996 through 1999 were revised using an approximation method for consistency with the revision to the 2004 and 2005 estimates.

[2]Implementation of Census 2000-based population controls occurred for the 2000 ASEC, which collected data for 1999. These estimates also reflect the results of follow-up verification questions, which were asked of people who responded "no" to all questions about specific types of health insurance coverage in order to verify whether they were actually uninsured. This change increased the number and percentage of people covered by health insurance, bringing the CPS more in line with estimates from other national surveys.

[3]The data for 1999 through 2009 were revised to reflect the results of enhancements to the editing process.

[4]Implementation of 2010 Census population controls.

Note: Respondents were not asked detailed health insurance questions before the 1988 CPS. The data points are placed at the midpoints of the respective years.

Source: U.S. Census Bureau, Current Population Survey, 1988 to 2012 Annual Social and Economic Supplements.

DEMOGRAPHICS OF ED PATIENTS

Most of the available data on emergency department visits comes from the *National Hospital Ambulatory Medical Care Survey* (NHAMCS). In 2009, the latest year for which data has been released, there were an estimated 136 million ED visits nationwide (compared to 95 million in 1997).[15] Notable observations include:

- Children under one year of age have the highest ED visit rates, followed by the elderly.
- Females visit at higher rates than males.
- Black/African-American patients visit at nearly double the rate of white and Hispanic patients; black patients aged 15-24 have the highest per capita visit rates of any demographic group (95.5 visits per 100 persons per year).
- Top chief complaints were, in decreasing order: abdominal pain, fever, chest pain, cough, headache, shortness of breath, and back pain.

COVERAGE STATUS OF ED VISITORS

Approximately 40% of ED visits are paid for by private insurance, 30% by Medicaid, and 17% by Medicare; 16% of patients are uninsured or self-pay.[15] Looking at per capita visit rates, Medicaid users visit at significantly higher rates (Figure 4), and their visit frequency appears to be trending upward. Between 1997-2007, ED visits by privately insured patients remained unchanged, and visits by uninsured and Medicare patients dropped. These statistics debunk the myth that emergency departments are filled with uninsured patients who are bankrupting the health care system.[17] In reality, the uninsured don't visit the ED significantly more than Medicare patients.

Visits by Medicaid patients, however, rose sharply by 36%. *Why* Medicaid patients visit the ED at significantly higher rates has been a long-debated topic in health policy circles.

Figure 4. ED Visits by Expected Source of Payment

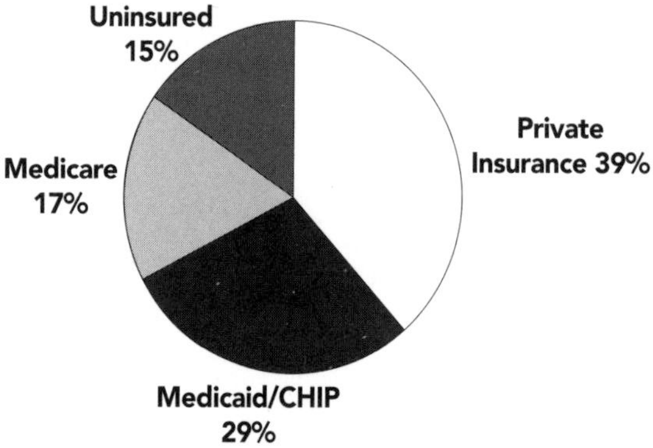

Uninsured 15%
Private Insurance 39%
Medicare 17%
Medicaid/CHIP 29%

Based on data from NHAMCS 2009.[15]

Studies have shown that Medicaid enrollees have reduced access to outpatient care.[18,19] Medicaid enrollees also are sicker than other patients; in fact, 29% of Medicaid enrollees are disabled. In surveys, only 31% of Medicaid enrollees report "excellent" or "very good" health, compared to 54% of the uninsured and 67% of privately insured. Still, researchers[20] report that – even when controlling for the differences in health status, demographics and socioeconomic status – half of the visit rate difference is unexplained. Furthermore, Medicare enrollees on average have more chronic diseases than Medicaid enrollees, yet visit the ED less than half as much.[20]

Medicaid visitors have lower rates of admission than the privately insured (9.5% vs. 14.1%; the Medicare rate is 33%),[15] but whether this reflects a higher rate of low-acuity visits by Medicaid patients is debated. Some suggest that the reduced admissions may be due to bias from admitting physicians. While Medicaid patients have a slightly higher rate of non-urgent visits (and a correspondingly *lower* rate of *emergent* visits) than privately insured patients, the vast majority of Medicaid visits are emergent, urgent or semi-urgent.[21] This is a complex and poorly understood problem; more research is needed to clarify the issue and propose solutions.

Figure 5. ED Visit Rates by Source of Coverage

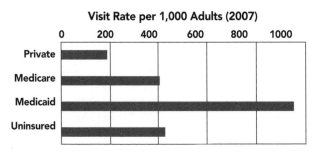

Based on data from Tang, et al, 2010.[16]

FREQUENT ED USERS AND SUPERUSERS

Every ED seems to have a socially marginalized (often alcoholic, homeless, or chronically ill) person who visits the hospital numerous times a month. These are the so-called *superusers*, also known as "highly frequent users"; they typically are uninsured[22] and visit the ED at extraordinary rates. But superusers represent just a small fraction of "frequent" ED users. While frequent users (often sick and elderly) only account for 4.5% to 8% of the total ED patient population, they account for 21% to 28% of all visits.[22] By contrast, superusers make up only a tiny percentage of total patients and account for an estimated 3.6% of ED visits.[23]

Most frequent users (the definition varies, but the most accepted definition is ≥ 4 visits/year) are, in fact, insured – usually publicly, with 60% insured by Medicaid or Medicare. Most are Caucasian (60%) and sicker than the average ED population.[22] Many hospitals are utilizing case management interventions in an attempt to reduce the number of emergency visits by frequent users and superusers. Studies of these interventions have shown mixed results, however.

AFFORDABLE CARE ACT AND ED VISITS

The coming years of health care reform and population demographic shifts promise to change the entire medical landscape significantly. With these changes, the emergency department (the canary in the coal mine of the U.S. health care system) likely will undergo major shifts in visitor patterns and demographics. The bulk of ACA reforms will take effect in 2014; as millions of people are added to Medicaid and private insurance rolls, the impact on emergency departments remains uncertain. If the new Medicaid *enrollees* visit at the same rate as current Medicaid *patients*, ED visits will rise rapidly.

Some have looked to Massachusetts, which enacted insurance reforms similar to the reforms of the ACA, to help predict how emergency department visits may change. Research on the aftermath of those reforms, however, found a small 4% rise in ED visits from 2006 to 2008, with a 2.6% decrease in low-acuity visits.[24] The rise in ED visits in Massachusetts (after reform) mirrored the rise in visits in neighboring states that did not enact any insurance expansion or reform.[21a]

One of the notable features of the Massachusetts reforms is a "public option" health plan known as *Commonwealth Care*. This plan requires copays for many services, including ED visits, for beneficiaries with incomes above a certain level.[25] Research on the use of cost-sharing to limit non-emergent ED visits has been limited and mixed. While initial studies in the 1970s suggested that copays could limit ED use, subsequent research has shown that copays do *not* have a significant impact on visit frequency. Some data also suggests that both emergent and non-emergent ED use may be reduced by copays, potentially endangering the health of patients and increasing long-term costs through increased morbidity and mortality.[23]

CONCLUSION

The U.S. health care insurance system is a complex tapestry that directly causes and affects patterns of resource utilization, including ED visits. The full impact of the ACA has yet to be seen and, given the complexity of the system, it is impossible to predict its full effects. Regardless, there will remain a substantial uninsured and underinsured population that will continue to challenge emergency departments and the system at large. ✶

Chapter 7

HEALTH DISPARITIES IN THE UNITED STATES

Kene A. Chukwuanu, MD

Health disparities have become a topic of increasing concern in recent years. With heightened societal interest in illuminating these inequities, it is imperative that medical professionals possess a clear understanding of the effects of social inequalities, their effects in creating and perpetuating health disparities, and their impact on the patients we serve.

While disparities, in general, have been classically presented in terms of race and ethnicity, the literature on disparities in *health* indicates differences within races, within and between income levels, with regard to places of residence, and within special populations. The social determinants of health also play a major role in individual and community health status. Health disparities are perpetuated by a large number of complex factors, including health insurance coverage, patient behaviors, quality and distribution of providers, and patient-provider interactions.

> *The wide gaps in health status among…marginalized populations is astounding. Righting the wrongs of these inequities should be both an ethical imperative and a matter of social justice for health care professionals.*

THE ECONOMIC BURDEN OF HEALTH DISPARITIES

The United States currently is spending more than $2 trillion annually on health care; this number is predicted to rise in coming years.[1] The impact of health disparities on total health care expenditures proves difficult to estimate.

Researchers estimate that greater than 30% of direct medical costs incurred by African Americans, Hispanics, and Asian Americans were attributable to racial and ethnic health disparities – an estimate of more than $230 billion over a three-year period from 2003 to 2006.[2] In addition, when indirect costs of these inequities – such as lost productivity, lost wages, absenteeism, family leave, and premature death – were tabulated, the total cost over the same three-year period was $1.24 trillion.[2] Given that people of color are estimated to account for more than half of the U.S. population in 2045,[3] it is imperative that the social inequities and their contributions to the health status of Americans be properly addressed.

THE SOCIAL DETERMINANTS OF HEALTH

According to the World Health Organization (WHO) Commission on Social Determinants of Health (CSDH),[4] the social determinants of health "are the conditions in which people are born, grow, live, work and age"; this also includes their health system. "These circumstances are shaped by the distribution of money, power and resources at global, national and local levels, which are themselves influenced by policy choices."[4] These determinants include social and environmental factors such as gender, race, living environment and housing, education, employment status, income, food availability and nutrition, and access to health care services and health insurance. Such determinants have been found to have the greatest impact in the propagation of health inequities.[4]

Given the great importance of these social factors, the WHO recommends confronting them by improving daily living conditions and addressing the inequitable distribution of money, power and resources. The organization also recommends the development of a workforce trained in social determinants in order to better measure and understand the problem and assess the impact of actions.[4]

The deep systemic problems driving health disparities will require broad policy solutions. Significant advocacy and community-building will be necessary to address these problems, as they exceed the scope of emergency care alone. As a safety net for the millions of Americans experiencing these disparities, emergency physicians are uniquely situated to provide powerful evidence of these dynamics and begin to address these issues on both individual and local levels.

DEFINING DISPARITIES

Many questions regarding the proper definition and classification of health disparities persist. What constitutes a disparity? What differences constitute a disparity? How many differences, and by what measure, are needed to equal a disparity? And, finally, when is it appropriate to label differences between groups with "the more politically charged term of a disparity?"[5] These are questions that many, both publically and privately, struggle to answer.

A *disparity* is *indirectly* measured, while *differences* can be *directly* measured; this contributes to the confusion regarding an appropriate definition of "health disparities." Though many federal institutions, national and international leaders, and private sector organizations have presented consensus statements and research surrounding access to and quality of care, they provide varying definitions of the term. Such differences contribute to confusion in the public sphere, increase the difficulty in assessment of inequalities in health status, and hinder the creation of policies to address them.[5]

WHO defines disparities as "differences in health which are not only unnecessary and avoidable but, in addition, are considered unfair and unjust."[6] This implies that unfairness in differences in health status constitutes disparities and is dependent upon choice, so that those who unwillingly exist in states of poor health due to measures beyond their control are those primarily afflicted.[5]

The groundbreaking 2003 Institute of Medicine (IOM) report on health inequality within the United States, *Unequal Treatment: Confronting Racial and Ethnic Disparities in Health Care*, defines health disparities as the "racial and ethnic differences in quality of care that are not due to access-related factors, preferences, and appropriateness of intervention."[7] In initially deriving this definition, the committee focused on disparities unrelated to access as charged by Congress. After further research, however, they concluded that such disparities only could be adequately addressed by first examining the problems related to health care access, behavioral risk factors, and socioeconomic inequalities.[5] The IOM report intentionally focuses on both health care system operations (and the legal and regulatory climate within which they function) and individual, patient-provider level discrimination.[7]

Since 2003, the United States Congress has required the Agency for Healthcare Research and Quality (AHRQ) to report on the opportunities for, and the progress of, improvements in health care quality and health disparity reductions; the results are published annually in the *National Healthcare Quality Report* and the *National Healthcare Disparities Report*.[8-9] The AHRQ was instructed to focus on "prevailing disparities in health care delivery as it relates to racial factors and socioeconomic factors in priority populations."[10] The AHRQ's definition of disparities seems to be the most specific and measurable, stating they are "any differences among populations that are statistically significant and differ from the reference group by at least 10%."[5,11]

Income Inequalities and Health Status

Socioeconomic status affects health status and health care access. Lower socioeconomic status is associated with decreased access to health care, limited community resources, increased risky health behaviors, higher levels of underinsurance and no insurance, and higher rates of mortality.[12] More significantly, when controlling for socioeconomic status, many health disparities are greatly reduced.[12]

A 2002 study examining income inequalities by U.S. counties found that those counties with increased inequalities in income had higher mortality rates.[13] Furthermore, African Americans have higher levels of income inequality and are more likely to have family incomes below 200% of the federal poverty level.[12-14] Controlling for individual income accounted for only one-third of the increase in mortality among black Americans. This may be due to the fact that many middle-income African Americans live in socio-environmental conditions that are consistent with a lower socioeconomic status.[13]

SPECIAL POPULATIONS

The Disabled

In 1990, President George H.W. Bush signed the Americans with Disabilities Act with the stated intent of bringing down "the shameful wall of exclusion."[15] As of 2011, 45 million people (19% of the country's non-institutionalized population) were living with some sort of disability. With that number expected to dramatically increase in the next 30 years as baby boomers age and retire, health care institutions will be challenged to provide adequate care for the nation's most vulnerable.

People with disabilities are increasingly disadvantaged in respect to the social determinants of health. They have been found to have lower educational levels, lower incomes, lower rates of preventive screening, higher rates of unemployment, and face increased difficulty in accessing health services than those without disabilities.[15] Those with disabilities also have higher rates of behavioral risk factors associated with poor health status, such as smoking, obesity, and inactivity; they also are significantly more likely to self-report fair or poor health than those without disabilities.[15] Physicians may contribute to poorer health in those with disabilities by failing to address risky behaviors in these populations. Additionally, the health care industry has struggled to provide the necessary services and equipment needed by those with disabilities, contributing to the substandard health care they receive.[15]

Rural Populations

Place of residence also has been studied as a contributor to the persistence of health disparities. A study in 2011 examined the health status and mortality differences of rural African Americans and rural white populations, as compared to *urban* whites. They found that excess mortality existed among residents of nonmetropolitan U.S. counties and was especially profound amongst rural African Americans.[16] Rural adults of all races "were more likely to characterize their health as "fair" or "poor" than were their urban counterparts,"[16] and reports of poor health were disproportionally higher among rural black and Hispanic individuals (39.6% and 30.4%, respectively). Additionally, rural residents were more likely to have been hospitalized during the past year.[16]

IMPLICATIONS OF HEALTH REFORM ON RACIAL AND ETHNIC DISPARITIES

Prior to the passage of the ACA, minorities constituted one-third of the U.S. population, but over 50% of the uninsured, with African Americans and Hispanics having much higher rates of uninsurance (21.6% and 33.3%, respectively) when compared to their white counterparts (13.9%).[3,17] Rates of health insurance coverage among all racial groups are expected to increase with the full implementation of ACA, with the greatest beneficiaries being among African Americans and Hispanics.[17] As insurance coverage expands, "reductions in long-standing racial and ethnic differentials in access and health status"[17] are predicted to follow.

Although governmental insurance programs will add many new minority enrollees, the most prevalent insurance type across all racial and ethnic groups will continue to be employer-based coverage. Among African Americans and Hispanics, the estimated rate increase of employer-based coverage is approximately 2.0% and 3.1%, respectively; among white Americans, who already have higher rates of employer-based coverage than all other groups, the increase is an estimated 0.9%.[17] Accordingly, the total rate of employer-based insurance after ACA implementation is a projected 65.6% for whites, 38.1% for African Americans, and 45.4% for Hispanics.[17] After implementation of the ACA, however, approximately 26.4 million people will remain uninsured, including a disproportionate number of African Americans and Hispanics (particularly undocumented immigrants).

DISPARITIES IN EMERGENCY MEDICINE

A large review of literature in emergency medicine, conducted by the Society for Academic Emergency Medicine (SAEM) as part of its 2003 consensus conference, documented significant health disparities in emergency medicine.[18] The organization found poorer outcomes – and higher rates of illness – among racial and ethnic minorities with emergency medical conditions such as chest pain and acute coronary syndromes, asthma, traumatic injuries, cancer mortality, strokes, and adequate analgesia, among others.[19-23]

In order to address these disparities, systems-based strategies were discussed, such as the increased use of evidence-based clinical guidelines to reduce the influence of stereotypes in clinical decision-making in emergency care, increased awareness of unconscious bias, education on cultural competency, improved patient-provider relationships, and increased workforce diversity.[22,24-26] In the years since this conference, more people have become uninsured; more people are utilizing emergency care;[27] and health disparities – which are difficult to identify and measure, and even more difficult to overcome – remain.

Although limited progress has been made in reducing health disparities, Americans are becoming increasingly aware of their existence. According to a 2010 survey, 59% of Americans "were aware of racial and ethnic disparities that disproportionately affect African Americans and Hispanics or Latinos."[28] This represents a modest increase from a similar 1999 survey, in which only 55% of Americans indicated their awareness of the problem; the same survey also revealed "low levels of awareness among racial and ethnic minority groups about disparities that disproportionately affect their own communities."[28]

Awareness of disparities appeared to be influenced by educational attainment; 55% of those with a high school education (at minimum) expressed awareness of racial and ethnic health disparities, compared to 36% of those who had not graduated from high school.[28]

CONCLUSION

The wide gaps in health status among minorities, the disabled, in rural communities, and in other marginalized populations within this country are astounding. In addressing these disparities and advocating for their reduction, unnecessary mortality is reduced and the health of the community and nation as a whole is improved. Righting the wrongs of these inequities should be both an ethical imperative and a matter of social justice for health professionals who have pledged to consecrate their lives to the service of humanity. ✱

Chapter 8

MEDICARE REIMBURSEMENT AND THE SUSTAINABLE GROWTH RATE

Harbir Singh, MD and Chet Schrader, MD

Medicare's *Sustainable Growth Rate* (SGR) was enacted in 1997 as part of the Balanced Budget Act in order to link annual updates of physician payments to the *gross domestic product* (GDP). It is intended to control the growth in Medicare expenditures for physicians' services. As medical costs have outpaced GDP growth, however, a crisis has arisen. Since 2003, Congress has had to intervene almost annually to eliminate cuts in Medicare payments for physicians.

> The SGR formula, with its inherent flaw of being tied to GDP instead of actual physician cost, has called for continued reductions in physician reimbursement in the face of rising practice costs.

PHYSICIAN VALUATION

In order to better understand how the SGR affects physician payments, it is important to first understand first *how* Medicare pays physicians. When a physician performs a service, that service is assigned a *relative value unit* (RVU). The determination of the "value" of an RVU is made by the Resource-Based Relative Value Scale Updates Committee (RUC), which designates an RVU to each CPT (billing) code (RBRVS). The RUC, which includes emergency physician representation, assigns the RVU for a service by taking into account three separate "values":

1. The value of the physicians work (WORK)
2. The value of practice expenses (PE)
3. The amount of professional liability insurance (PLI) for the particular service

It is important to recognize that any change in valuation of services must be "budget neutral." In other words, any increase in the value of one service will result in an equivalent decrease in the value of another service. There is a finite amount of federal money distributed through the RUC procedure; new spending in one area must be offset by cuts in another area. As a result, an *increase* in reimbursement for one physician/specialist results in the *decrease* in reimbursement for a different physician/specialist.

Each RVU is then adjusted for differences in reimbursement throughout the country by a *geographic practice cost index* (GPCI). Finally, the entire RVU is multiplied by a conversion factor (CF), which assigns an actual dollar amount to the payment a physician receives.

The final Medicare physician rate formula is:

Medicare Physician Payment = CF x [(RVU$_{WORK}$ x Budget neutrality adjustor x GPCI$_{WORK}$) + (RVU$_{PE}$ x GPCI$_{PE}$) + (RVU$_{PLI}$ x GPCI$_{PLI}$)]

Each year the dollar amount allocated to the conversion factor is adjusted. To calculate the change, the Center for Medicare & Medicaid Services (CMS) takes into account two factors:

Medicare Economic Index (MEI)
Measures the cost of resources needed to provide physician services
Designed to estimate the increase in the total cost for the average physician to operate a medical practice
Update Adjustment Factor
Based on the comparison of spending for services subject to the SGR and the formula's target spending
Accounts for spending in a given year and that year's target budget and the relationship between cumulative spending and the cumulative target budget

SGR CALCULATION

According to CMS, the sustainable growth rate is calculated based on the estimate of the change in each of four factors. The four factors for calculating the SGR are:

1. The estimated percentage change in fees for physicians' services.
2. The estimated percentage change in the average number of Medicare fee-for-service beneficiaries.
3. The estimated 10-year average annual percentage change in real gross domestic product per capita.
4. The estimated percentage change in expenditures due to changes in law or regulations.[1]

The SGR initially was developed with the goal of controlling Medicare spending on physician services. Essentially, legislation dictates to CMS that the SGR will cut payments to control spending if growth in Medicare patients' use of services exceeds the growth in GDP. It is important to clarify, however, that the change in gross domestic product reflects neither the change in patients' health care needs nor the cost for a physician to run a practice. The cost of utilization of services can increase if Medicare changes coverage policies; technology is implemented that allows patients access to new – albeit more expensive – treatments; or more patients are enrolled in Medicare, as is expected with the aging baby boomer population.

The SGR formula, with its inherent flaw of being tied to GDP instead of actual physician cost, has called for continued reductions in physician reimbursement in the face of rising practice costs. Thanks to ACEP, the American Medical Association, and other physician organizations, these cuts have been temporarily averted numerous times. Since 2010, the law has required four extensions with lapses of up to 20 days after expiration and processing of actual payment cuts. With each temporary fix, the debt owed to the SGR increases and, consequently, the cost of the next predicted reduction gets exponentially larger.

In February of 2012, President Obama signed the Middle Class Tax Relief and Job Creation Act of 2012, which further delayed the implementation of the conversion factor until January 1, 2013, avoiding an estimated cut of 27.4%. This amendment is the 14th patch the SGR has required over a 10-year time period. Yet another one-year delay was passed on January 1, 2013; at press time, an approximate 30% cut is scheduled for January 1, 2014.

FUTURE SGR REDUCTIONS

A 2007 Medicare Trustees Report predicts a total reduction in Medicare physician payment rates of approximately 41% over the next nine years as a result of the flawed SGR formula,[2] while the cost of running a practice and caring for patients is expected to increase by nearly 20%.[3] In addition, a 2005 Medicare Payment Advisory Commission (MedPAC) survey found that "25% of Medicare patients looking for a new physician had some problem finding one."[4] With impending cuts and rising costs of practice, it is expected that physicians will continue to turn away from treating Medicare patients. In fact, according to a 2006 AMA survey, "67% of physicians say they will decrease or stop seeing new Medicare patients if the scheduled eight years of cuts take place."[4]

SGR SOLUTIONS

Traditionally, Congress has acted only to provide a series of short-term fixes; recent efforts to provide a permanent fix to the SGR have failed. The Deficit Reduction Act of 2005 mandated that MedPAC examine alternative mechanisms for controlling physician expenditures, and, more specifically, configure ways to reformulate the SGR. Since then, MedPAC repeatedly has released reports recommending alternatives to the sustainable growth rate.[5,6] The commission's most recent reports indicate that the SGR has failed to restrain volume growth, and that the frequent fixes are "undermining the credibility of Medicare" with providers and patients.[7a]

ACEP, the AMA, and other physician organizations have continued to press Congress to work towards a permanent solution. Proposed ideas include:[7b]

1. Changing the SGR and tying growth to the MEI rather than the GDP
2. Changing it to a GDP +x% model
3. Creating service-specific updates (or "buckets"), such as separate SGR formulas for anesthesia; evaluation and management services; imaging and tests; major procedures and minor procedures
4. Eliminate the SGR and replace it with a long-term stable schedule of fee updates. MedPAC has been recommending this since 2011.[7a,7b]

SGR EXCLUSION FROM REFORM

Early in the health care reform debates, Congressional leaders decided that an SGR fix would not be included; instead, they opted to introduce concurrent legislation to provide a permanent fix. Unfortunately, despite lobbying efforts by ACEP and other physician organizations, the Senate defeated Senate Bill 1776 – which would have repealed the SGR and frozen current reimbursement rates – by procedural vote. Additionally, the House introduced HR 3961, which would have repealed the current SGR and replaced it with a new formula that creates two updates: GDP +2 for evaluation and management services and GDP + 1 for other services. Initially, it passed in the House by a largely partisan 243 to 183 vote, but was stripped of the SGR fix by Senator Harry Reid via a "manager's amendment" in the Senate. With an estimated cost of more than $350 billion for a permanent solution,[7b] Congress has been unable to identify a funding source for a long-term remedy and, instead, has opted to provide only a series of short-term fixes.

THE INDEPENDENT PAYMENT ADVISORY BOARD

In an effort to address the challenge of controlling Medicare costs, Senate leaders introduced one of the more controversial components of the Patient Protection and Affordable Care Act – the creation of the Independent Payment Advisory Board (IPAB). The 15-member IPAB is a presidentially appointed board consisting of health care and economic experts, whose responsibility it is to provide specific proposals to reduce Medicare spending in years where spending is determined to exceed an initially pre-set target growth rate (initially based on the *Consumer Price Index*). IPAB members are not required to be physicians, a seemingly significant oversight.

Beginning in 2013 the IPAB will make cost-reduction recommendations to Congress and the President; if Congress fails to pass the IPAB's recommendations or come up with its own alternative legislation to reduce spending, the Department of Health and Human Services *must* implement the IPAB's spending reduction strategies.

While initial estimates from the Congressional Budget Office predict that the IPAB will yield a reduction in Medicare spending of approximately $28 billion from 2010 to 2019,[8] significant concerns remain about the board's effectiveness. For example, rate reductions for hospitals and hospices explicitly are excluded until 2020. Additionally, IPAB cannot make recommendations that limit eligibility, increase premiums, or limit coverage (i.e., "ration health care"). Given these restrictions, the IPAB has few alternatives to control costs, other than cutting reimbursement to providers.

In a detailed report, the CMS actuary noted that IPAB target growth rates only would have been met *four* times in the last 25 years, and these target growth rates would look similar to the SGR – a flawed formula that has been consistently overridden by Congress.[9] With many impending reimbursement reductions, the CMS actuary expressed concern that health care providers would leave the Medicare program, compromising access to care for seniors and other Medicare beneficiaries.

CONCLUSION

Until a new system is implemented, the sustainable growth rate will remain an annual threat to physician income, patient access to care, and the long-term viability of the Medicare system. The high price tag of reform and the impending exhaustion of the Medicare Trust in 2029[10] present immense challenges. As bills are brought forward to propose new ideas for physician reimbursement and alternatives to the SGR, detailed evaluation and advocacy for appropriate reform will be required. While physicians wait for long-term reform, annual update legislation will require strong support and aggressive advocacy to prevent catastrophic cuts in reimbursement. ✷

Chapter 9

NEW METHODS OF PAYMENT: VALUE-BASED PURCHASING AND EPISODES OF CARE

Michael Dorrity, MD and Seth Trueger, MD

In an era of increasing health care expenditures with no apparent limits in sight, cost effectiveness is fast becoming a necessity. The current system of fee-for-service payment is often criticized for rewarding *quantity* rather than *quality* of care. This system has been likened to a homeowner paying an electrician for each outlet installed, and then wondering why he ended up with a kitchen full of outlets.

We are a privileged nation with a high volume of health care, but many would argue that we are not much healthier for it. A 2012 Institute of Medicine Report estimates that 30% of health care spending ($750 billion) is wasteful, stemming from unnecessary care; missed opportunities for preventative care; errors; fraud; and administrative, economic, and operational inefficiencies.[1]

The trend among payers (the Centers for Medicare and Medicaid Services [CMS] is the biggest) is to become *active*, rather than *passive*. CMS and other payers are beginning to link *quality* to *payment* through various means, including bundling payments to cover episodes of care; pay-for-performance; and developing health care delivery organizations that align payment incentives with longitudinal patient outcomes *(patient-centered medical homes)* and community outcomes *(accountable care organizations)*.

VALUE-BASED PURCHASING

One of the concepts touted by CMS is *value-based purchasing* (VBP). Since CMS policies have the power to transform the health care system as a whole, the hope is that private insurers will follow the organization's lead by adopting VBP to help improve quality and contain overall growth in health care costs.

Major goals of VBP

Financial viability	Maintaining Medicare's solvency
Payment incentives	Linking payments to value (quality and efficiency)
Joint accountability	Providers accountable for care in their communities
Effectiveness	Evidence-based and outcome-driven care
Ensuring access	Equal access to high-quality, affordable care
Safety and transparency	Where beneficiaries receive this information
Smooth transitions	Coordinated care across different providers and settings
Electronic health records	Where information technology supports providers

More than a specific program, VBP is an over-arching concept that CMS is using to guide and shape the way it pays hospitals and providers. The goal is to restructure the fee-for-service system by implementing projects, programs and demonstrations, using VBP principles as a guide.[2] The mechanism for this implementation has been incremental, but implementation is aggressively accelerating.

One program central to VBP in hospital care is the CMS *Hospital Value-Based Purchasing Program* (HVBP). Authorized by the ACA and beginning with hospital discharges in October 2012, CMS will adjust FY2013 Medicare payments to hospitals based on their relative performance on a range of quality metrics for the care of acute myocardial infarction, heart failure, pneumonia, surgical procedures, hospital-acquired infections, and the Hospital Consumer Assessment of Healthcare Providers and Systems (HCAHPS) patient satisfaction survey.

HVBP is phased in over time; by 2017, hospitals will see an increase or decrease in up to 2% of their overall Medicare reimbursements, as determined by these quality and patient satisfaction scores.[3] Similarly, the ACA established the *Hospital Readmission Reduction Program* (HRRP), which will reduce overall Medicare payments to hospitals by up to 3% if their 30-day readmission rates for acute myocardial infarction, heart failure, or pneumonia exceed targets.[4]

EPISODES OF CARE AND BUNDLING

Payment bundling refers to a single payment made to cover all services related to a given treatment or condition. Government and private payers, as well as some providers, are incorporating bundled payments under the concept of *Episodes of Care* (EOC), with the goal of decreasing costs and improving quality and efficiency. An EOC can be defined as "the total cost of hospital services, physician services, and other services required for treating an acute condition" or, alternatively, as "the total cost for all the care required during a given year for a patient with chronic conditions."[5] The idea is that payers would allocate one lump sum for each EOC to be distributed between facilities and providers, either for all of the care involved in a hospitalization and follow-up, or for treating a chronic condition for an entire year. Examples include surgical procedures with one payment given to cover pre-op, surgery, anesthesia, post-op care, and follow-up visits.

Under the Affordable Care Act, Medicare will start paying for some surgical procedures with a bundled EOC payment.[6] Further, the ACA established the Center for Medicare and Medicaid Innovation within CMS in 2011 to "test, evaluate and expand" different payment structures and methods within programs run by CMS, many of which are piloting demonstration projects with EOC payment structures. This will include EOC built around acute care (defined as beginning three days prior to admission and extending to 30 days following discharge), as well as chronic condition EOC through both Medicare and Medicaid.[7,8]

It is important to differentiate *bundled payments* and *coordinated care delivery* (e.g., ACOs). Whereas EOC results in a single lump payment to a hospital for *all* the care surrounding a surgical procedure, coordinated care delivery models – such as ACOs – "bundle" a patient's care under a network of providers; elements of that care, however, still may be paid for based on a fee-for-service model, with the providers sharing in any savings obtained through care coordination.

It is not clear yet how emergency physicians will fit into these new models of payment. As emergency physicians sit at the nexus of hospital readmission and other targets of bundling, there is a potential for inclusion in a lump sum payment to a hospital or other care organization, which would then divide out payments to the various providers. The risk to emergency physicians is that they will be negotiating individually with powerful groups that may work to reduce physician reimbursement. If payments are made to hospitals, which then distribute them among providers, one could envision a hospital underpaying physicians to maintain its bottom line or directing money toward specialties seen as revenue-generators. Alternatively, this may push more hospitals to employ emergency physicians directly to avoid these negotiations and simplify recordkeeping. As a result, the potential exists that many of the improvements in reimbursement and physician autonomy that we have developed as a specialty may disappear if these programs are not implemented in a fair and balanced way. It is unclear how emergency care and reimbursement will fit into EOC, but there are concerns that emergency physicians will be pressured to provide less care for patients when faced with these restrictions.[9]

Even with the passage of the Affordable Care Act, the consequences remain uncertain; there will be political hurdles to implementation. It is imperative that emergency physicians get involved *now* to influence future programs and regulations. ACEP has passed a resolution committing to work with CMS to develop demonstration and pilot projects for new payment models and remains active in the legislative and regulatory processes involved in health care reform.[10]

Are There Problems With This Kind of Payment?

The underlying assumption in VBP and EOC is that physicians will change their practices based on financial incentives and that these changes eventually will improve the quality of health care. The idea of value-based purchasing makes great sense on the surface. We all make value judgments every time we make a purchase and want the most for our money; the problem is deciding *who* defines that value and *how* it should be defined. For most daily economic activity, the individual making the purchase and receiving the service defines value in their own terms. In health care, third-party payment has changed this interaction. While patients naturally want the best available care, they're rarely forced to consider the cost, since someone else is paying the bill. The challenge of VBP will be defining *value* in ways that are good for individual patients, while being economically and financially feasible for payers and providers.

Further, the overall impact of the Affordable Care Act on total health care expenditures remains to be seen. While the ACA includes many cost-saving measures and efforts to streamline delivery and improve the quality of care, major provisions also expand coverage and access to care. Improved efficiency therefore may be offset by increased quantity as more patients seek care; the ultimate effect on overall health care costs is yet to be seen.

CONCLUSION

The movement toward VBP and EOC appears to be gaining support; indeed, CMS already has implemented aspects of both. Regardless of the merits of the system, it inevitably will impact the practice of emergency medicine, both financially and professionally. Clinicians need to be involved in establishing how VBP is implemented, how EOCs are defined, and how payments are distributed to ensure that incentives remain appropriate and patient-centered.

Some would argue that physicians passively stood by while business people, lawyers, and politicians established the policies that govern how physicians work. As the providers of America's health care safety net, emergency medicine physicians are in a unique position to speak to the downstream effects of current and future payment and policy decisions. Changes in payment structure will have significant effects on our pocketbooks, on our patients, and on the quality of care that we provide. ✳

Additional Resources

- Centers for Medicare & Medicaid Services: Quality Initiatives: http://www.cms.gov/QualityInitiativesGenInfo
- Hospital Value-Based Purchasing: http://www.cms.gov/Medicare/Quality-Initiatives-Patient-Assessment-Instruments/hospital-value-based-purchasing/index.html
- American College of Emergency Physicians: Resources on Episode-Based Reimbursement: http://www.acep.org/bundledpayments

Chapter 10

MEASURING QUALITY IN EMERGENCY MEDICINE

Daniel Stein, MD, MPH

INTRODUCTION

Emergency departments and emergency physicians across the country are standing in a brighter spotlight than ever before. Recent national tragedies (mass shootings, acts of terrorism, natural disasters) and ED crowding continue to attract the attention of the media and regulatory agencies alike. Emergency departments increasingly are being viewed as the "front door" to the hospital; with more than 136 million annual visits,[1] Americans are being evaluated in EDs in record numbers. With this escalating visibility and utilization comes an increased responsibility to ensure that the quality of care we provide our patients remains uncompromised.

"We want to make sure that we incentivize the health care system to be designed to provide you the best quality health care possible."
— Valerie B. Jarrett, Senior Advisor to President Barack Obama, Chair of the White House Council on Women and Girls

The medical community has long been aware of the challenges emergency physicians face when delivering quality medical care. In the 1960s and 1970s, physicians began examining adverse events in hospitalized patients. Many of these events were the result of human error;[2,3] further research confirmed that many of these errors were *preventable*.[4,5] Two reports published by the Institute of Medicine (IOM) in 1999 and 2001, *To Err is Human* and *Crossing the Quality Chasm,* responded to these studies. The IOM called upon the health care system to focus on six specific "Aims for Improvement" – safe, timely, effective, efficient, equitable, and patient-focused care.[6] Then, in 2006, the Institute of Medicine published *The Future of Emergency Care,* in which it recommended "convening a panel with emergency care expertise to develop evidence-based indicators of emergency care system performance."[7]

As a unit, these three reports changed the way health care providers and hospitals viewed patient care. Perhaps more importantly, they changed the way both the public and the government viewed the health care system. The public began to understand *quality* as a critical piece of determining its value.[8] These realizations translated into important changes in how – and on what – health care dollars are spent; quality improvement became aligned with performance measurement and patient-centered care.

ENTITIES IN DEVELOPING QUALITY METRICS

Determining evidence-based quality measurements that are clinically meaningful, attainable, and cost-effective is a challenging process. Any individual or organization can submit quality measures to the Centers for Medicare and Medicaid Services (CMS) or the Physician Quality Reporting System (PQRS) for consideration. Submissions have been considered from a broad range of interest groups, including medical specialty organizations, patient advocacy groups, and nonprofit health care organizations. There are a few large organizations, however, that place a heavy emphasis on developing and submitting evidence-based quality measures.

National Quality Forum (NQF)

NQF may be the single largest player in standardizing measures for health care quality, and serves as a clearinghouse for national priorities and goals for system-wide improvement. Historically, it has served as the final common pathway for quality measure endorsements; CMS has generally adopted many of the measures endorsed by NQF.

Physician Consortium for Performance Improvement (PCPI)

The American Medical Association sponsors the PCPI, a national, physician-led program focused on developing evidence-based performance measures for the health care system. Anyone interested in health care quality can join; however, full voting members must be representatives of physician organizations (AMA, AOA, state chapters, specialty organizations, medical boards, etc.). The PCPI has authored 280 performance measures that encompass nearly every field in medicine.

National Committee for Quality Assurance (NCQA)

The NCQA is a not-for-profit organization known for publishing the *Healthcare Effectiveness Data and Information Set* (HEDIS). HEDIS is designed to allow health consumers to compare health plan performance with regional and national benchmarks that can be categorized into the following areas of quality measures: effectiveness of care, access and availability of care, experience of care, utilization and relative resource use, and health plan descriptive information. NCQA also offers accreditation and certification programs for various entities, including accountable care organizations, new health plans, physician organizations, and health information products.

PHYSICIAN QUALITY METRICS

The Physician Quality Reporting Initiative (PQRI) was launched by CMS in 2007 as part of the Tax Relief and Health Care Act of 2006 with the goal of linking physician quality with payment incentives. In 2007, PQRI began with 74 quality measures. It offered an initial 1.5% payment bonus to those physicians who successfully participated in the program, with a subsequent increase to 2% bonus payments in 2009 and 2010. The Affordable Care Act made adjustments to PQRI; it became the Physician Quality Reporting System (PQRS), signaling a shift from the quality metric being an exploratory initiative to a large, comprehensive system.[9] ACA expanded the metric and required the formation of an appeals process and the ability to provide physicians with timely feedback. In 2011, CMS finalized payment adjustments to those physicians who participated successfully in PQRS. Payment gradually will be adjusted from a 0.5% bonus incentive in 2012 to a 2% payment rate penalty in 2016 and beyond, based on the previous year's performance.[10,11] (Table 1)

Table 1. PQRS Incentive Payment Structure

Year	PQRS Incentive Payment Adjustment
2012	+0.5%
2013	+0.5%
2014	+0.5%
2015	-1.5%
2016+	-2.0%

PQRS is not specialty-specific; *any* physician may report on *any* quality measure. A list of PQRS measures that generally are believed to affect emergency physicians is included here (Table 2). Physicians are required to report on three metrics in any given year and are eligible for the additional bonus (2012-2014) or are immune from the payment penalty (2015 and beyond) if they comply at a specified rate (50%-80%).

Here is a brief example:

*You are treating a 28-year-old woman for abdominal pain in the emergency department. In your work-up, you order a urine pregnancy test and document the order and the result. Your coding and billing agency will give you credit for quality measure #253 (pregnancy test for female abdominal pain patients). If you do **not** order the pregnancy test and document **why** you did not order the test (for instance, the woman is 36 weeks pregnant), you would still get credit for reporting on that quality measure. If you do this for at least 50% of female patients presenting with abdominal pain and also for at least two additional quality measures, you would be eligible for the incentive.*

Table 2. PQRS Quality Measures Relevant to Emergency Physicians[10]

PQRS #	Quality Measure
28	Aspirin at arrival for acute myocardial infarction (AMI)
31	Stroke and stroke rehabilitation: deep vein thrombosis prophylaxis (DVT) for ischemic stroke or intracranial hemorrhage
54	12-Lead electrocardiogram (ECG) performed for non-traumatic chest pain
55	12-Lead electrocardiogram (ECG) performed for syncope
56	Community-acquired pneumonia (CAP): vital signs
57	Community-acquired pneumonia (CAP): assessment of oxygen saturation
58	Community-acquired pneumonia (CAP): assessment of mental status
59	Community-acquired pneumonia (CAP): empiric antibiotic
76	Prevention of catheter-related bloodstream infections (CRBSI): central venous catheter (CVC) insertion protocol
91	Acute otitis externa (AOE): topical therapy
92	Acute otitis externa (AOE): pain assessment
93	Acute otitis externa (AOE): systemic antimicrobial therapy – avoidance of inappropriate use
252	Anticoagulation for acute pulmonary embolus patients
253	Pregnancy test for female abdominal pain patients
254	Ultrasound determination of pregnancy location for pregnant patients with abdominal pain
255	Rh immunoglobulin (Rhogam) for Rh-negative pregnant women at risk of fetal blood exposure

HOSPITAL QUALITY METRICS

Quality metrics are contextualized for care settings; to reflect this, *inpatient* metrics are differentiated from *outpatient* metrics. Emergency departments (considered outpatient care) straddle the setting gap between outpatient and inpatient care and are substantially affected by hospital operations; emergency physicians should be aware of these dynamics, as hospital policies are often influenced by the hospital quality reporting system.

Hospital care quality is measured by five generally accepted factors, which payers – including CMS – use to determine the quality of hospitals. Quality performance, through the Hospital Inpatient Prospective Payment System (IPPS) and Outpatient Prospective Payment Systems (OPPS), directly affects the hospital's CMS reimbursement rates. Critical access hospitals and certain rural hospitals are exempt from this reporting system. The five factors that determine hospital quality are:

- Patient experience (as measured by HCAHPS, the national metric for grading hospitals)

- Process quality (whether hospitals are adherent to evidence-based guidelines)
- Mortality rates (proportion of people who die within 30 days of hospitalization, taking into account the "sickness" of the patient)
- Readmission rates (proportion of people who are readmitted within 30 days of discharge, taking into account the "sickness" of the patient)
- Hospital safety score (a measure of how effective a hospital likely is at preventing medically-induced harm to patients)

Process quality is reported using both the Hospital Inpatient Quality Reporting System (IQR) and the Hospital Outpatient Quality Reporting System (OQR), depending on the context within which care is delivered. There are a number of outpatient measures that are reported based on health care quality in the emergency department (Table 3). While there are a number of parallels between the physician and hospital quality metrics, they are measured independently of each other. Although hospital adherence to these measures directly affects hospital reimbursement rates, they do not affect physician reimbursement.

Table 3. Hospital OQR Quality Measures Relevant to Emergency Departments[12]

OP#	Hospital OQR Quality Measures
OP-1	Median time to fibrinolysis
OP-2	Fibrinolytic therapy received within 30 minutes of ED arrival
OP-3	Median time to transfer to another facility for acute coronary intervention
OP-4	Aspirin at arrival
OP-5	Median time to ECG
OP-12	The ability for providers with HIT to receive laboratory data electronically
OP-14	Simultaneous use of brain-computed tomography (CT) and sinus CT
OP-15	Use of brain CT in the emergency department for atraumatic headache – **UNDER REVIEW**
OP-16	Troponin results for emergency department acute MI or chest pain patients within 60 minutes of arrival – **SUSPENDED***
OP-17	Tracking clinical results between visits
OP-18	Median time from ED arrival to ED departure for discharged ED patients
OP-19	Transition record with specified elements received by discharged patients – **SUSPENDED**
OP-20	Door to diagnostic evaluation by a qualified medical professional
OP-21	ED-median time to pain management for long bone fracture
OP-22	ED-patient left without being seen (numerator/denominator one time per year for designated reference period)
OP-23	ED-head CT scan results for acute ischemic stroke or hemorrhagic stroke who received head CT scan interpretation within 45 minutes of arrival

*Suspended due to concerns about use of point-of-care troponin assays that have poorer test characteristics than laboratory-based troponin assays.

CONTROVERSIES IN QUALITY MEASURES

The development of quality measures that affect both patient care and reimbursement rates has spurred much controversy. The lack of evidence required to support each measure and the potential errors in implementation that may occur when the original proposed metric is misapplied are particularly troubling.

There are three major issues unique to emergency medicine that have raised concerns over the program:

Outpatient Measure 15 (OP 15): CT Scans of Atraumatic Headache.

Despite NQF rejection, CMS has an imaging efficiency measure currently under review, which addresses the use of brain CT scans in the evaluation of atraumatic headaches in emergency departments. The measure calculates the percentage of ED visits by Medicare beneficiaries for headache with a coincident brain CT study. The stated goal is to encourage judicious use of brain CT scans in patients with uncomplicated headaches; a lower number of CT scans is considered to be superior. There are some important exclusion criteria intended to isolate uncomplicated headaches (for example, headache associated with lumbar puncture, dizziness, paresthesia, lack of coordination, complicated or thunderclap headache, focal neurologic deficit, pregnancy, HIV, tumor or mass, or CT scan related to reason for admission).

Data published in 2012 indicates that OP-15 is not a reliable, valid, or accurate way to assess emergency department performance.[13] Researchers reported numerous cases in which OP-15 deemed a CT scan *inappropriate* when it likely was warranted, according to ACEP's clinical guidelines or expert consensus. One example was that of a 67-year-old male patient with a known brain aneurysm, who was sent to the ED by his primary care provider because of concern for a subarachnoid hemorrhage (SAH). The emergency physician ordered a brain CT and did a lumbar puncture to rule out SAH, but the brain CT was labeled inappropriate because the lumbar puncture was not properly coded. These types of measures raise serious concerns that physicians will be pressured to deviate from the standard of care based on billing guidelines — putting patients and themselves at risk.

Outpatient Measure 19 (OP 19): Transitions of Care.

Studies of care between the various settings in the health care system have shown that there are substantial patient safety and quality inadequacies in the way our system currently manages *transitions*.[14] In 2009 ACEP, SAEM, and other specialty organizations published a consensus statement that called for accountability; clear communication with patients, their families, and providers taking over care; and the establishment of national standards for transitions in care.[15] Emergency departments often are not properly equipped to manage these transitions, predisposing patients to poor outcomes. ACEP's Transitions of Care Task Force recommended, among other things, improving residency training in transitions, developing and evaluating successful transition systems, and assessing provider performance with appropriate feedback.[16]

CMS established OP 19 to encourage emergency departments to provide discharged patients with a detailed transition record that includes major procedures and tests performed during any ED visit, principal diagnosis or chief complaint at discharge, patient instructions, plan for follow-up care, and a list of new medications and changes to continued medications. Because of hospital concerns about the current specifications and privacy issues, the measure was suspended in 2012.[17] This measure is likely to be reviewed in the future and may return with some revisions.

Public Reporting of Quality Measures. The 2006 Tax Relief and Health Care Act, while establishing PQRI (now PQRS) as the incentive payment program for reporting data on quality measures, also required the creation of a physician quality reporting system. Launched in 2013, the CMS *Physician Compare* website publicly reports information on physicians and other eligible professionals who participate in the Physician Quality Reporting System. Information reported must include data on the quality measures collected, as well as assessments of patient health outcomes, risk-adjusted resource use, efficiency, patient experience, and other relevant information deemed appropriate by the HHS secretary. Physicians will have a reasonable opportunity to review their results before the information is made public.

Though this level of transparency generally is well-regarded by health care consumers and physicians alike, challenges loom on the horizon. Determining how to adequately maintain the site, keep information interpretable to consumers, and assess its relevance in emergency medicine are issues that will need to be addressed. Currently, physicians are given an unlimited amount of time to review their results, so it is difficult to keep the site updated. In general, patients cannot *choose* their emergency physicians, which makes the system's applicability to the specialty questionable. Perhaps, most importantly, it is impractical and ill-advised for a patient to consult the Medicare website to find the "best" physician while having a heart attack, stroke, or other acute medical emergency.[18]

> *"For patients, their families, and their care providers, sifting through complex and disparate diagnostic, and therapeutic information to agree on a unified plan of care is problematic. At the least, we waste time trying to decide what is important and actionable. At the worse, we fail to execute transitions of care successfully, and then we increase costs, diminish quality, and increase the likelihood for adverse outcomes."*
> – ACEP Transitions of Care Task Force Report

CONCLUSION

Quality metrics in emergency medicine are here to stay; as an emergency physician, your reimbursement will be based — at least in part — on your ability to adhere to the standards that have been developed by various groups. You should familiarize yourself with the quality metrics that have been developed and launched into the PQRS and OPPS in recent years. This controversial system, while seeking to increase both the quality and value of medicine, has many limitations. Provider-based and hospital-based quality measures will affect clinical care, timeliness of care, emergency department throughput, hospital and physician finances, and resource utilization issues. The trend in linking adherence to quality metrics and payment are likely to continue in *Episodes of Care* measures, which are based on value-based purchasing and bundled payments. ✱

Chapter 11

NEW HEALTH CARE ORGANIZATIONS

Kevin Blythe, MD

Effective quality primary care is at the core of the world's highly efficient medical care systems; it provides services that positively impact the overall health of a population, usually at a fraction of the cost of more specialized care services. The lack of comprehensive, organized primary care in the United States frequently is cited as one of the reasons that our country has fallen behind other nations in many health quality indicators, despite extraordinarily high national spending on health care.[1] In recent discussions about health care reform, policy makers have sought solutions to the imbalance between *primary* and *specialty* care, with the expectation that improvements in primary care will result in both decreased health care costs and improved patient outcomes. *Patient-centered medical homes* (PCMH) and *accountable care organizations* (ACO) are two concepts that have been touted as capable of delivering such results.[2]

THEORY OF PCMH

The basis of the PCMH is centrally coordinating medical care under a single primary care provider, thus eliminating the inefficiencies and hazards of multiple specialists individually managing aspects of a patient's health. Special emphasis also is placed on encouraging the PCPs to utilize technological advancements and evidence-based quality improvements to increase the quality and efficiency of care – additionally allowing patients greater access to their providers. The American Academy of Pediatrics (AAP) describes the care provided by PCMHs as "accessible," "continuous," "comprehensive," "family-centered," "coordinated," "compassionate," and "culturally effective."[5]

HISTORY OF PCMH

The PCMH certainly is not a new idea. The term "patient-centered medical home" first was introduced in 1967 by the AAP to describe a structure whose purpose it was to centrally organize pediatric medical records for children with complex medical conditions.[5] The concept of the PCMH was later redefined by the American Academy of Family Physicians (AAFP), which extended the scope of medical homes to include the provision of coordinated, comprehensive primary care for a patient's entire lifespan. In 2007 a consortium of primary care providers comprised of the AAP, AAFP, American College of Physicians (ACP), and American Osteopathic

Association (AOA) defined the medical home as: "an approach to providing comprehensive primary care for children, youth and adults. The PCMH is a health care setting that facilitates partnerships between individual patients and their personal physicians and, when appropriate, the patient's family."[6] The consortium also provided seven key principles to define the concept:

- **Personal physician.** Patients have access to a personal physician with whom they can develop a continuous ongoing relationship. These personal physicians will provide first contact, and continuous and comprehensive care.

- **Physician-directed medical practice.** The personal physician will take lead of a team of individuals which will collectively take responsibility for the ongoing care of patients.

- **Whole person orientation.** The personal physician will take responsibility for providing *all* of the patient's health care needs or appropriately arranging care with other qualified professionals. This responsibility encompasses all stages of life and all states of health.

- **Care is coordinated and/or integrated.** Care is facilitated by health information technology and exchanges across all elements of health care systems (e.g., subspecialty care, home health, nursing homes) and community services. Indicated care is to be provided to the patient, when and where it is needed or wanted, in a culturally and linguistically appropriate manner.

- **Quality and safety.** Practices ensure quality of patient care and experience via several methods: adoption of evidence-based medicine and clinical decision tools to support decision-making, participation in performance measurement and quality improvement, and utilization of information technology to support patient care. Physicians encourage active patient participation in decision-making and performance management to ensure that the patient's expectations are being met.

- **Enhanced access.** Access to a patient's personal physician is made more readily available through techniques such as open scheduling, expanded office hours, and utilization communication technologies (e.g., e-mail).

- **Payment.** Provider reimbursement is appropriately adjusted for the added value provided to patients in a PCMH. Payment should include fee-for-service payments for office visits, but also reflect the value of additional services provided, including: coordinating care with other providers, extending access to care, and adopting and utilizing health information technology. Physicians should share in the savings related to reduced hospitalizations and receive additional payments for achieving measurable quality improvements.

EARLY RESEARCH RESULTS

Theoretically appealing to providers, policy makers, and patients alike, the PCMH concept has been promoted by several provisions in the ACA and implemented in various-sized pilots around the country with promising results.[3] Pennsylvania's Geisinger Health System yielded a 7% reduction in total medical costs in the first year of implementing a PCMH model, while simultaneously improving patients' experiences.[7] Similarly, the Community Care of North Carolina system self-reports an annual savings of $20-25 per patient three years post-adoption of a similar model.[8] These two pilots demonstrate that anticipated benefits can be achieved given the right circumstances; however, other studies have not proven as promising.

The *Patient-Centered Medical Home National Demonstration Project*, which examined 36 family practices transitioning to PCMH models over a two-year period, did not find any improvement in patient health status, satisfaction with service, coordination of care, or comprehensiveness of care, despite significant adoption of PCMH model components among the studied practices.[9] A different study, which analyzed health costs over a five-year period for primary care practices with varying levels PCMH adoption, found that increased PCMH component adoption led to decreased costs *only* in the most medically complex group of patients. Total costs increased for patients in the low and medium complexity groups.[10]

Analyses of the costs associated with PCMH adoption show that a significant investment is required for measurable improvement in practice operations.[3] PCPs may eventually reap the benefits of improved practice organization; however, with no guarantee of long-term profits, the initial investment may be cost-prohibitive for independent and hospital-associated practices.[11] Many of the projects that have demonstrated an effective transition to the PCMH model have benefitted from an already integrated health system with a pre-existing infrastructure and resources to facilitate the transition.

MOVEMENT TOWARD STANDARDIZATION

While many of the goals of the PCMH have been outlined, details about adoption, implementation, and quality assurance have yet to be clearly defined or standardized.[2] In a survey of PCMH implantation projects across the country, researchers discovered a "wide-spectrum" of pilots in scope, design, and methods of evaluation.[11]

In an attempt to reduce the wide variability amongst practices, the National Committee for Quality Assurance (NCQA) developed a set of standards for evaluating PCMHs. As of 2011, more than 1,500 practices have gained PCMH recognition by adopting those standards. It has been noted, however, that the NCQA standards do not completely align with the seven principles detailed by the patient-centered primary care collaborative, with uneven weight placed on technologic improvements versus the assurance of comprehensive and coordinated care. [2] With other organizations creating their own competing criteria, it is clear that further work in the development and evaluation of PCMH standards is necessary.

IMPACT ON EMERGENCY MEDICINE

While emergency medicine is not directly addressed by the PCMH model, a broad reorganization of primary care could affect how patients utilize the ED, change the role of emergency medicine physicians in coordinating care, and impact physician compensation. Early analysis has suggested that some PCMH patients had a significant decrease (up to 29%) in the number of ED visits.[12] Most financial analyses on the impact of PCMHs has focused on savings related to this decrease in emergency department utilization and inpatient admissions.[3] This data, however, should not be used to diminish the critical role of emergency medical care within any health care system nor implicate emergency departments in the rapid expansion of the health care costs. In fact, the CDC estimates that emergency departments *serve more than 136 million Americans annually, while accounting for only 2% of medical costs.*[13]

PCMH adoption does not address the more than 50 million Americans who are currently uninsured and depend on emergency departments to provide safety-net care. With these facts in mind, it is critical for ED reimbursement to remain uncompromised in the face of primary care restructuring. In 2008, ACEP released a statement regarding PCMHs, in which it affirmed its support of efforts to improve primary care in the U.S.

ACEP cautioned against haphazard redistribution of limited health care resources – the practice of taking from one critical sector of health care to bolster another. In the policy statement, ACEP stressed the unique and vital role of the emergency department as a safety net for the un- or underinsured, as required by EMTALA. The organization highlighted eight issues that must be addressed with widespread implementation of PCMHs:[14]

- ACEP supports high-quality, safe, and efficient medical care.
- ACEP supports health care payment reforms that ensure all medical providers are fairly compensated for the care they provide to patients.
- Enhanced access must be demonstrated.
- Once established, the medical home should continue regardless of insurance status or ability to pay.
- Patients must have freedom to switch medical homes, select specialists of their choosing, and access emergency medical are when they feel they need it.
- Research must prove the value of the medical home before it is widely adopted.
- Universal health insurance coverage is necessary for the PCMH model to be most effective.
- The medical home must include the safety net of emergency care.

These issues pose a number of implementation challenges for patient-centered medical homes that have not been fully addressed. Before widespread implementation, it will be critical for emergency physicians to advocate for patients throughout their care spectrum and, in particular, when they may need to access emergency services.

ACCOUNTABLE CARE ORGANIZATIONS

Accountable care organizations (ACO), in conjunction with PCMHs, have been touted as a means to curb health care spending. The core element of ACOs is a network of providers who take financial responsibility for providing high-quality, cost-effective care. As envisioned when the term was first described in 2005, a PCMH-like primary care practice takes the lead in providing patient care and coordinating with other providers as needed.[16] A provider-led case reviewing organization reviews the quality of care provided by an individual practice and distributes bonus reimbursement from a "shared savings pot," created from the savings reaped through cost-effective measures. Reimbursements are based on provider performance in meeting quality care objectives.[15-16] Improvements in health information technology are stressed, with the goal of accurately monitor provider performance. Improvement in EMRs results in better patient care and allows ACOs to efficiently monitor achievement of health care objectives.[17]

ACOs reform traditional payment schemes (fee-for-service and capitation) to reward measurable quality improvement and cost-effective care. Historically, fee-for-service models may have encouraged providers to see a great *quantity* of patients at the expense of *quality* care. The new system will shift these incentives; for example, CMS guidelines for ACOs participating in a Medicare pilot program scored providers on categories including coordination of care and the caregiver experience.[17] These important aspects of patient care are discouraged in fee-for-service models.

Physicians receiving capitation payments are not under the same pressure to maximize patient volume; however, they may sacrifice quality of care by limiting services rendered to increase profits. Capitation also encourages "cherry-picking" of generally healthy (and thus, less expensive to treat) patients, decreasing access to care for the most at-risk patient populations;[2] CMS accountable care organization guidelines include measures to guard against these abuses. In fact, almost half of the total measures outlined relate to providing care to the elderly and patients with diabetes, heart failure, coronary artery disease, hypertension, and COPD.[17]

PROMISING EARLY RESEARCH RESULTS

In 2006, Blue Cross Blue Shield of Michigan initiated a program to enhance primary care by providing financial incentives for physician groups to make improvements in the coordination of care and patient communication, and to develop better patient registries.[16] After five years of implementation among a group of 8,000 PCPs, analyses showed savings via 2% lower radiology usage, 1.4% lower ED usage, and 2.6% lower adult inpatient admissions.[16] In addition, $19 million was saved in the two years following implementation of standards to increase generic drug use.[16] Blue Cross Blue Shield of Massachusetts launched a program in 2009, in which providers received incentives for measurable patient experience and outcome objectives through a modified fee-for-service system. In the first year of the program, all participants produced a year-end surplus that was reinvested in practice infrastructure improvements.[16] Compared to controls, participants had three times better scores in preventative care measures; patients also were found to utilize the ED for non-emergent issues less often.[16]

CHALLENGES TO ACCOUNTABLE CARE ORGANIZATIONS

There are substantial challenges to implementing an accountable care organization. *Primary care physicians* are the central figures within an ACO model. Currently only 35% of physicians, 37% of physician assistants, and 50% of nurse practitioners work in primary care fields.[18] Already acknowledging a shortage of PCPs, research shows that physicians may need to work 3.2 additional weeks per year to coordinate care for medically complex patients under these new models.[19] Large investments in health information technology and infrastructure improvements may be prohibitive to smaller practices.[2] There also is sure to be public push-back against any reform that would limit the freedoms currently enjoyed by patients, who likely will resist giving up their ability to refer themselves to doctors of their choosing.[19]

CONCLUSION

The patient-centered medical home concept has been proven successful in small trials, leading some to believe that the model might improve the problem of America's strained primary care system. Accountable care organizations, too, have exhibited promising results in isolated trials and have been promoted by the ACA as a means to decrease health care costs and improve patient care. Neither concept, however, has been proven cost-effective, beneficial, nor practical on a national level. Current systemic deficiencies of primary care in the U.S. may be prohibitive to successful implementation. As emergency medicine physicians, increasing access to quality primary care will result in improved quality of life and outcomes for our patients. Implementation of such improvements should not be made haphazardly, however, nor come at the expense of the health care system's safety net or its providers. ✴

With thanks to Kelly M. Doran, MD for her authorship of a previous version of this chapter.

Chapter 12

BALANCE BILLING

Nadia Juneja, MD

Balance billing refers to the practice of physicians billing patients for additional charges not paid for by their health care plans due to the physician being labeled "non-contracted" or "out-of-network." The crux of the problem lies in determining fair payment for services provided in the absence of a *prior agreement* between physicians and insurance companies. Although this process impacts all aspects of health care, it is particularly problematic in the emergency department, where patients seldom choose their providers and physicians are mandated (under EMTALA) to provide care to *every* patient, regardless of insurance status. As emergency physicians increasingly serve as safety-net providers, ensuring fair payment from insurance companies is of significant importance to guarantee continued access to care.

AN ISSUE OF FAIR PAYMENT

The underlying problem of balance billing lies in determining fair payment for services provided when no prior agreement has been established between physicians and insurance companies. When these parties disagree on fair payment, the insurance company may decline to provide full payment for what has been billed by the physician and then bill the patient for the remaining charge. Currently, there is no agreed upon guideline accepted by both parties to determine fair payment for a given service.

CONTRACTUAL ANOMALY

The debate on fair payment and the practice of balance billing arises in non-contracted or out-of-network care for insured patients.* In the setting of functioning contracts, providers have agreed to accept a given rate for their services and patients do not experience balance billing.

For example, if a physician sets his or her fee at $100, that will be the amount billed. If the physician provides care to an uninsured patient, that patient will be billed $100 (although this may never be collected). If the physician provides care to a privately insured patient, and the physician is an "in-network" provider for that insurance company, the physician may instead accept a reduced fee – for

---

*In this chapter, "insured patients" refers to patients insured by managed care organizations; "insurance companies" is intended to designate managed care organizations. Many preferred provider organizations are also held to the same rules and provisions as discussed; however, other insurance policies such as self-insurance may not apply.

example, $80 – for that same service. The physician is agreeing to accept $80 as *full payment*—as well as consenting to the overall fee schedule determined by the insurance company. The division of the responsibility for payment between the insurer and the patient is based on the insurance company's contract with the patient, but does not change the total payment, even in the setting of co-pays or deductibles.

However, if the physician provides care to a privately insured patient and is not an "in-network" provider for the patient's insurance company, the fee submitted remains $100. Every individual insurance company may establish a set amount as reimbursement for each service. If a patient is seen by an out-of-network physician, for example, the fee may be $100; the insurance company, however, will only reimburse the physician $80, in keeping with the insurance company's previously established reimbursement for that service. If the physician then bills the patient for the remaining $20, this is an example of balance billing.

UNIQUE CHALLENGES IN THE ED

Outside of the emergency department, physicians may establish contracts with insurance companies of their choice. When a physician believes the reimbursement or other policies of an insurer are unfair or undesirable, they may elect not to contract with that company. Physicians are not required to contract with specific companies or accept patients with specific coverage. Patients are aware of the financial consequences if they choose an out-of-network physician; these consequences are explained in their insurance coverage statement of benefits. The statement usually will include a list of covered providers, which may include emergency physicians.

In the context of a medical emergency, however, patients should be focused on receiving rapid, high-quality medical care, not on finding an *in-network* emergency department or emergency physician. Unlike physicians who provide elective and scheduled care, emergency physicians do not check their patients' insurance status before treatment – a practice that would raise ethical concerns, impede the provision of timely emergency care, and violate our federal mandate to provide emergency stabilization to all patients under EMTALA.[1]

Given the legal requirement to provide care for all patients, emergency physicians cannot turn away those who are out-of-network. After providing care, emergency physicians believe they should be reimbursed appropriately based on the reasonable and customary value of their services. Emergency physicians already provide the most uncompensated care of all physicians in EMTALA-related bad debt; ensuring fair payment from insurance companies is of significant importance.[2] As a result, emergency physicians may balance-bill patients to ensure fair compensation for care.

FEDERAL REGULATIONS ON BALANCE BILLING

In 2010 the Patient Protection and Affordable Care Act was passed, providing the first federal regulations on balance billing. Provisions in the law introduced requirements for coverage of emergency services, precluding the need for prior authorization or increased cost-sharing for emergency services, whether provided by in-network or out-of-network providers.[3] The act of balance billing was not directly prohibited in the bill.

Interim final rules published by the Department of Health and Human Services (HHS) took effect in 2010 and require coverage for emergency services without prior authorization or benefit limitations based on whether providers are in or out of network. HHS also specifies minimum payments for out-of-network providers to prevent increased cost-sharing on the part of plan beneficiaries.[4] Set minimum benefits for out-of-network providers are equal to the greatest of three possible amounts:

1. the median in-network provider rate
2. the amount for the emergency service calculated using the same method the plan generally uses to determine payments for out-of-network services (such as the usual, customary and reasonable charges)
3. the amount that would be paid under Medicare.[5]

The regulations' minimum payment standards were developed to protect patients from financial penalties related to the use of emergency services on an out-of-network basis. By setting minimum payment standards, HHS ensured plans would not pay an unreasonably low amount to an out-of-network emergency service provider, resulting in the patient being balance billed.[6]

Although intended to protect the insured, there is concern the rules may have significant *unintended* consequences. As written, the rules allow insurance plans to dictate usual and customary rates; many believe that this power should be placed in the hands of an independent board, given the inherent bias of insurance companies seeking to minimize their expenditures. Because the Medicare rate already is highly discounted, this leaves physicians with very little leverage to negotiate a fair payment. Similarly, as in-network providers accept lower rates to account for the other benefits included in their contracts, it would be unfair to require non-contracting physicians to accept the same discounts with no additional benefits.

> *Emergency physicians have few physician allies in legislative battles about balance billing, as we are uniquely obligated by EMTALA to see all patients, regardless of our relationship with their insurance networks.*

These rules were created to protect insured patients from increased cost-sharing, but fail to address the underlying dispute regarding fair payment and offer no incentives for insurance companies to reimburse physicians at fair market rates. These unresolved issues may instead increase the discordance between charges and reimbursement, leading to increased balance billing.

Furthermore, in states where balance billing has been prohibited or if a plan is contractually responsible for any amount balance billed by an out-of-network provider (as in a "hold harmless" clause), the plan is not required to meet the payment minimums. While patients are protected with adequate notice to prevent inadvertent payments on their part, this leaves no protection against an unreasonably low reimbursement rate for out-of-network physicians.[7]

USUAL, CUSTOMARY AND REASONABLE CHARGES (UCR)

Prominent in the debate surrounding compensation for out-of-network services is the insurance industry's use of *usual, customary and reasonable* (UCR) charges for determining reimbursement. Prior to 2009 the majority of insurance companies utilized one of two national databases, both owned by Ingenix, which compiled data to determine the UCR rate for a particular service in a given area.[7] Prompted by complaints regarding Ingenix's practices, in 2008 the company underwent extensive investigation by New York State Attorney General Andrew Cuomo.

Results of the investigation determined the company held an inherent conflict of interest as a wholly owned subsidiary of UnitedHealth Group; in addition, rates generated by Ingenix data were often discounted by as much as 30% below actual market rates.[9] New York State's action and multiple class-action lawsuits from medical societies across the country filed against United and other major carriers led to the closure of Ingenix. In addition, United pledged to spend $50 million to help establish a new independent database to be governed by a nonprofit agency, FAIR Health, Inc. (Fair and Independent Research).[7]

FAIR Health was created in October 2009 with a mission to serve as an independent, objective and transparent source of health care reimbursement for consumers, insurers, health care providers, researchers, analysts and policymakers.[11] Its database launched for insurers, physicians, and consumers in 2011; one year later, it was opened for use in academia to promote public health research on spending and utilization.[12]

Although the settlements led United and other insurance companies to provide the monetary means to create FAIR Health, the companies never admitted guilt and have no requirement to utilize the organization's database in determining their own charges. In what has been described as an effort to avoid increased reimbursements and use of the FAIR Health database, many insurance companies have shifted toward reimbursement based on a percentage of Medicare rates.[13] In the 2011 New York state legislative session, a bill was passed that required a minimum payment for out-of-network services to be set at a percentage of actual charges, based on the FAIR Health database; the bill was later recalled, however, and remains in assembly at this time.[14]

It is still too early to determine whether FAIR Health will be more reliable than the Ingenix database it replaced, or how widely the database will be utilized. With no current standards accepted, charges designated as "usual, customary and reasonable" can be, in many instances, ambiguous – a problem that remains a frequent topic of policy debate.

STATE REGULATIONS ON BALANCE BILLING

Some states have policies designed to prevent balance billing by removing the patient from the dispute between providers and insurers. In most instances, this is achieved by requiring insurance contracts to include *hold harmless provisions,* or provisions releasing patients from liability to settle any balance bill received.[13] The intent is to force insurers to negotiate fair payment with providers, rather than leaving physicians with no other option than to balance bill. Nine states have gone further by *prohibiting* balance billing, including California, Delaware, Florida, Indiana, Maryland, New York, Rhode Island, West Virginia and Wisconsin.[14] Individual state policies vary widely, however; most either dictate appropriate reimbursement by limiting physician charges or by requiring insurers to pay billed amounts.

In Colorado, where hold harmless provisions are required, insurers are essentially mandated to reach agreement with providers on fair payment.[7,15] There is no specific law prohibiting balance billing; however, any patient who receives a balance bill is asked not to pay it.[7] Since the patient must be held harmless, insurers typically pay the billed charges or negotiate with the provider for a lower rate.[7] If any disputes regarding appropriate reimbursement are not resolved, they may be arbitrated at a later time. Insurers argue against such arrangements; they maintain that providers should not have full discretion to set their own charges and that payment of full charges will disincentivize providers from contracting with companies.[7]

In states where balance billing is prohibited, various strategies to designate payment rate requirements have been utilized; unfortunately, they all lack clear and objective definitions of the rate requirements. In California and Florida, appropriate rates are designated as either the "reasonable and customary value" or "usual and customary provider charges."[7] Neither defines how these rates shall be determined, however, leaving providers vulnerable to the insurance companies' interpretations of such guidelines.

Given the insurance industry's inherent bias and prior experience with attempts to unfairly reimburse, emergency physicians are concerned about regulations that prohibit balance billing without a process to negotiate fair payment. In states with such policies in place, physicians are left with little recourse to challenge payment decisions. Arbitration procedures have proved largely unsuccessful and require significant time and financial resources on the part of the physician.[7]

Balance billing and determination of fair payment continues to be an active issue in many states. In 2010, the Illinois legislature passed a bill including provisions to prohibit balance billing, which was later vetoed by the governor. In 2011 the National Conference of Insurance Legislators (NCOIL) adopted model legislation on out-of-network balance billing written with input from many medical societies, including ACEP. The main focus of the legislation is *transparency* and *notification of possible cost-sharing to patients*, rather than the prohibition of balance billing. In 2011 alone, seven states introduced legislation focused on out-of-network compensation, with legislators in Illinois, New Mexico, New Jersey and Indiana discussing possible prohibition or limits on balance billing.[7,18] These states are the latest – but not likely the last – targets of the movement to ban the practice.

FUTURE CHALLENGES

Until there is an agreed upon method for determining fair payment, emergency physicians will need to advocate for reasonable legislation on federal and state levels. Emergency physicians have few physician allies in legislative battles about balance billing, as we are uniquely obligated by EMTALA to see *all* patients, regardless of our relationship with their insurance networks. It is critical for emergency physicians to be aware of the legislative activities in their states and work to advocate for their patients and the specialty when issues of fair payment arise. Additionally, emergency physicians will need to remain active in regulatory advocacy as additional rules are established and revised to allow the implementation of health reform. ✶

Chapter 13

GRADUATE MEDICAL EDUCATION FUNDING

Puneet Gupta, MD and Erin E. Schneider, MD

In many ways graduate medical education (GME) funding is the lifeblood of emergency medicine; it keeps residency programs solvent to be able to produce residency-trained emergency medicine physicians. Despite this critical need, GME is under attack – chiefly because of significant financial challenges to Medicare, the largest contributor to GME funding. In the face of serious fiscal problems, the 113th Congress may implement major changes to our country's Medicare program. Emergency medicine health advocates already are hard at work to protect GME funding and provisions for residency-trained emergency physicians.

GME FUNDING: THE BASICS

Graduate medical education funding primarily is provided by the federal government through a variety of payers. The federal Medicare program, via the Centers for Medicare & Medicaid Services (CMS), contributes the majority of GME funding. The U.S. Department of Veterans Affairs (VA) separately funds 9% of all graduate medical education. The degree to which private insurers fund training-related costs is difficult to calculate, as GME payments are often included in patient care revenue.[2] Costs generally are divided into *direct* medical education (DME) and *indirect* medical education (IME).

Direct costs include resident salaries, overhead, and faculty supervision. DME costs are calculated based on a hospital's direct GME costs per resident, multiplied by the number of full-time equivalent residents and the number of inpatient days allotted to Medicare patients.[3] DME costs per resident for each institution were developed based on those incurred in 1984 or 1985, adjusted for inflation, and vary widely across the country; they are paid by patient services revenue from Medicare, Medicaid, the VA and private insurers.[4] Medicare spent about $6.5 billion in IME and $3 billion in DME in 2010.[5] In 2009, Medicaid payments to IME and DME totaled $3.8 billion.[6]

IME payments are justified by increased costs to hospitals associated with training residents and students. Academic centers have higher acuity patients, added staff, inefficiencies secondary to having multiple learners, and increased technological costs. The American Association of Medical Colleges (AAMC) reports that teaching hospitals "make up 20% of the nation's hospitals yet conduct almost two-thirds of the most highly specialized surgeries, treat nearly half of all specialized diagnoses, train almost 100,000 resident physicians and supply more than 70% of the hospital care provided to the nearly 43 million uninsured patients."[7]

IME is calculated based on the intern-and-resident-to-bed ratio. Given the difficulty in accounting for costs directly, IME has been the target of funding reductions in the past. Medicare IME payments were $6.5 billion in 2008, comprising a substantial percentage of GME funding. The IME equation calculates payments to teaching institutions using a multiplier determined by the U.S. Congress.[8]

This multiplier is based on the assumption that the inpatient operating cost per case is increased by a certain percentage with each 10% increase in the number of residents per hospital bed. The multiplier initially was set at 11.59%, based on recommendations from the secretary of the Department of Health and Human Services (HHS), then later reduced to 7.7% in 1997 when data on actual costs became available. However, CMS estimates that operating costs only increase 2.7% for every 10% increase in the resident-to-bed ratio, based on 2003 data. The Balanced Budget Act (BBA) of 1997, as well as subsequent legislation, set up annual reductions in the IME formula that reflected this and reduced the multiplier to 5.5% by 2003;[9] the current rate remains at 5.5%. MedPAC estimates the multiplier to be even lower (2%), based on its cost analysis from 2004.[3]

Disproportionate share hospital (DSH) payments are another funding source allocated to hospitals caring for a higher percentage of uninsured or underserved patients. The Medicare Prescription Drug, Improvement, and Modernization Act of 2003 allowed for a reduction in the cap on DSH payments to qualifying hospitals from 5.7% to 12% of total payments; payment adjustments of up to 25% are provided for low-volume hospitals (fewer than 800 total discharges per year) that are 25 miles or more from another hospital.[10]

EMRA Policy on Securing GME Funding for Resident Education

"EMRA will support current research and studies aimed toward revising current Graduate Medical Education funding mechanisms and work to change current Direct Medical Education regulations that limit research and extramural educational opportunities.

EMRA will work with other healthcare organizations to better define the problem of Graduate Medical Education funding and propose alternatives and solutions that may involve both the public and private sectors.

EMRA opposes reductions in Medicare funding for Graduate Medical Education at the Federal and State level and supports diversified sources of funding that help meet the overall goals of residency training."

Original policy adopted by Resolution Council, 5/08[1]

RESIDENT POSITION ALLOCATIONS

The Balanced Budget Act of 1997 placed a cap on the number of FTEs (residency spots) that CMS would fund, based on the number of residents a teaching hospital reported in 1996.[11] At the time it was predicted that there would be a *surplus* of 80,000 physicians by the year 2000. A number of CMS-funded unfilled residency positions were redistributed; rural and small urban areas picked up more CMS-funded positions in the redistribution. Multiple emergency medicine programs were awarded positions from their institutions and either started or expanded their residency programs. ACEP aided in this process by advocating for new criteria in the process of vying for positions. Approximately 26,772 residency positions have been added since 1995; most of them have been "above the cap," using different sources of revenue, including scholarships, endowments, and state support.[12,13]

The Affordable Care Act of 2010 (ACA) established a number of provisions that will affect GME funding if implemented. These include reducing the current cap on residency positions by 65% of currently unused slots (e.g., if six slots remain unused, the cap is reduced to two), with 75% of new slots going to primary care or general surgery (§5503). Unused slots from hospitals that close (§5506) also are redistributed, a rule that was implemented in 2011. The CMS revised the regulations (§413.79) in 2012, stating that any hospital receiving a §5503 grant would be evaluated from July 1, 2011 (the date of implementation) to July 1, 2016. At that point, any unused funding would be reallocated elsewhere.[14]

Further changes to the law during the process of implementation are expected.[14,15] Overall, the impact is likely to aid in expanding rural and off-site rotations, redistributing unused positions, and increasing primary care positions. Regardless, a shortage of 62,900 physicians is predicted by the year 2014; this situation will continue to worsen unless significant changes in residency funding are made.[16]

OUTSIDE ROTATIONS

While emergency medicine residency programs seek to increase training opportunities, a risk of financial penalty exists when rotations occur off hospital grounds. The Direct Graduate Medical Education (DGME) section of the Social Security Act, states:

> *"A hospital may count residents training in non-hospital settings for direct GME purposes... if the residents spend their time in patient care activities and if... the hospital incurs all, or substantially all, of the costs for the training program in that setting..."*[17]

These costs include salary, benefits, and costs of teaching staff. Outside hospitals that are approved by CMS teaching facilities may collect direct GME from CMS when a resident completes an outside rotation there. The primary residency may then request reimbursement from the outside hospital to pay salaries and benefits. Non-hospital settings, including non-teaching facility rural hospitals or other sites that may provide a key component of emergency residency training (i.e., poison control centers, pediatric centers), will not receive compensation from CMS because the hospital does not incur "all or substantially all" of the training costs. In this case, neither hospital receives compensation. Such a policy is a disincentive to the development of rural emergency medicine rotations and other non-hospital-based training opportunities; it also limits rotations in community settings that do not meet criteria to collect money directly from CMS.

DECREASING MEDICAID SUPPORT

A 2009 survey conducted by the AAMC noted that 41 states, plus the District of Columbia, contribute to DME/IME payments, down from 47 states in 2005.[5] Through the federal regulatory rule-making process, in 2007 CMS proposed to eliminate "inappropriate" payments from Medicaid to hospitals as a match to state funding.[18] This proposal would have hurt residencies in states that depend on this pool of money to fund graduate medical education. Initially extended to 2009, the moratorium on any action by the secretary of the U.S. Department of Health and Human Services (HHS) to restrict Medicaid payments for graduate medical education has been extended indefinitely. This issue may continue to arise and threaten GME funding as major reforms to health care are proposed.

DEFICIT REDUCTION COMMITTEE TARGETS GME

The Joint Select Committee on Deficit Reduction (the "Super Committee") was formed in 2011 to create a plan for long-term reduction in federal spending over the next 10 years to address the federal deficit. In the process of deliberation, Medicare reimbursement for GME was identified as a potential area of savings.[1a,19] The plans for savings are diverse and involve multiple organizations. MedPAC recommended decreasing indirect medical education spending from 5.5% to 2.2%, with a goal of using the surplus money for performance-based hospital incentive programs.[20]

The National Commission on Fiscal Responsibility and Reform (also known as the Simpsons-Bowles Commission) is a bit more radical; it recommended allocating an extra 3.3% to the federal government, rather than returning it to the hospitals.[21] The Congressional Budget Office (CBO) wants to eliminate the direct and indirect medical education systems altogether and, instead, provide a lump sum equating to 2.2% IME budget *plus* the DME budget *plus* $500 million – an approximation of Medicaid's federal contribution. The funds would be distributed based on the number of residents and inpatient days for Medicare/Medicaid patients, and would be adjusted annually for inflation. In addition, President Obama's budget calls for a reduction in IME spending from 5.5% to 4.95% beginning in 2014.[22]

Many groups, on the other hand, advocate for an *increase* in funding for graduate medical education, including EMRA and ACEP. A coalition of legislators introduced a bill in the 112th Congress that would increase the number of

Medicare-funded residency slots by 3,000 a year from 2013 to 2017 to address the impending physician shortage.[15] The legislation failed to pass in 2012, but was reintroduced in both the House and the Senate on March 15, 2013 – a day also known to residents and medical students around the country as "Match Day."[23] At press time, the future of the current bill is uncertain.

CONCLUSION

Despite any upcoming congressional action, ongoing advocacy will be necessary to ensure adequate graduate medical education funding. There are many advocacy opportunities for emergency medicine residents in the area of GME, including nationwide efforts to maintain Medicaid support and prevent further reductions in IME payments. With the implementation of the Affordable Care Act, it has become increasingly important for emergency medicine residencies to be recognized as a crucial part of graduate medical education. We anticipate GME funding challenges to escalate as the Medicare program becomes increasingly stressed. As the physician shortage continues to worsen, as well, continued advocacy for emergency medicine training will remain a critical component of attracting the best and brightest to the specialty. ✱

Chapter ✦ *14*

CURRENT CHALLENGES IN STUDENT LOANS

Katherine Nacca, MD

The cost of graduate education and the ensuing loan debt is an escalating struggle for nearly every medical student in the United States. In 2009, the vast majority of medical students (85.2%) graduated deeply in debt. Rising faster than inflation, the average debt burden now topples $145,000 (with an additional $10,000 for private schools) – a substantial increase from 2005, when medical school debt averaged $113,412.

In addition, the *pre*-medical school loan indebtedness of graduating young physicians averages $157,990. To compound matters, 33% of students carry an average $17,000 in *non-educational consumer debt*. The ever-rising cost of education has made it nearly impossible for students to graduate without significant loans[1]; simply put, most medical school students hold *some* amount of debt. This growing financial burden is of great concern for future health care professionals and individual medical specialties alike.

> *The rising cost of medical education is a heavy burden for resident physicians and has become an influential factor in the migration of medical students to more lucrative specialties.*

TYPES OF LOANS

There are several types of loans available to physicians-in-training, the most important of which are offered by the federal government. These loans frequently provide the lowest interest rates, an important factor that adds to their appeal.

Stafford loans are the primary loans available to medical students through the federal government. Until 2012, both *subsidized* and *unsubsidized* loans were available. Recent amendments to the Budget Control Act, however, eliminated subsidized loans for graduate education; subsidized loans granted prior to the amendment are not affected.

Subsidized loans were based on need and did not accrue interest until repayment of the loan began. Unsubsidized loans are *not* need-based; they begin to accrue interest during medical school and continue to compound that interest throughout the life of the loan with a fixed interest rate of 6.8% through 2013. $20,500 can be borrowed in Stafford loans annually, with a previously subsidized maximum of $8,500. Health professionals are eligible to borrow up to $138,500; the limits, however, are woefully inadequate in the face of current education costs.

Stafford loans may be supplemented by the use of private loans or *Grad PLUS loans*, which are backed by the federal government.[2] Like private or unsubsidized loans, Grad PLUS loans are not need-based. These loans offer a higher interest rate of 7.9%; the maximum borrowing amount equals the cost of attendance *minus* any other financial aid, including Stafford loans. Grad PLUS borrowers also pay an additional 4% in fees associated with disbursement.

If a student has a poor credit history or has incurred costs that surpass these loan amounts, additional *private loans* may be necessary. With interest rates typically much higher than those of federal loans,[3] however, bank loans are less desirable. Low starting "promotional" interest rates may have initial appeal – particularly in light of the recent ban on subsidized loans – but private loan interest rates are variable and inevitably increase to a higher average than those of fixed Stafford loans. The country's ongoing national financial crisis also has made these "high-risk" loans more difficult to obtain.

Need-based *Pell Grants* are available for some graduate students, but they typically are available only to those in *significant* financial need, with the goal of encouraging higher education for low-income Americans.

REPAYMENT ISSUES

There are several factors to consider when evaluating the repayment terms of loans: *grace period, deferment, forbearance*, and *consolidation*. Post-graduation, students are given a six-month grace period, during which no loan payment is required. Subsidized loans do not accrue interest during this time; other types of loans do. It is important to note that students who have taken loans *prior* to medical school and who have previously consolidated their debt may not be granted this grace period; payment may be required immediately after graduation, with interest accruing on all loans.

Resident physicians may begin to repay the loans after the six-month grace period, or may attempt to *defer* or *forebear* their loans. Deferment is a period during which no payment is required, but interest accrues (with the exception of the now-eliminated subsidized loans). This was a very popular option for resident physicians for many years; given their current low salaries, however, deferment is no longer widely available. Unemployment, severe economic hardship (including participation in the Peace Corps), and active military duty are conditions under which a deferment may be granted. Most resident physicians not enrolled in the military no longer fit into these categories. Of note, deferment is granted at some institutions in conjunction with fellowship, due to a legislative loophole.[4]

The most common repayment path for resident physicians is *forbearance*. This means that the borrower is responsible for the interest accrued on all loans, including those that are subsidized, but is not required to make payments on the loan. Forbearance may be granted for a maximum of three years. While it is useful to delay repayment of loans during residency, this option is less than optimal given the significant buildup of interest accrued during this period.

As a third option, resident physicians may begin to repay their loans immediately after medical school graduation. *Standard* repayment requires monthly payments on the loan to cover interest and a portion of the original loan. *Graduated* or *income-based* repayment options also are available, in which the monthly payment is set to increase over a certain time period or is based on the borrower's income. In addition, an *extended* repayment option is available for up to 30 years. It is important to keep in mind, however, that the interest continues to build on the loan regardless of its terms; the longer a borrower takes to pay it back, the higher the total amount paid.

Loan interest rates are a particularly important consideration. It often is difficult for a medical school graduate on a resident's salary to make payments on loans, leading many to seek forbearance. If it *is* possible to make payments, the borrower should focus on those loans with the highest interest rates, which will accrue interest the fastest.

INCOME-BASED REPAYMENT PROGRAM

The *income-based repayment* (IBR) *program* requires repayment to begin when the physician is able to make minimal payments based on a formulaic calculation that takes into account all students with debt. This program replaces the *20/220* plan that previously had exempted many residents from making payments during residency.[5] The goal of the program was to limit the amount of debt and encourage prompt repayment, an objective that ignores the economic realities of many residents. A minimal payment of even just a few hundred dollars can constitute a true hardship for struggling residents, particularly those living in expensive locations.[6]

In an attempt to ease the burden and increase awareness of available options, the Obama Administration introduced a memorandum designed to facilitate a simpler, streamlined process for IBR enrollment. Online resources and awareness of repayment options also were increased. Prior to the memorandum, very few borrowers – perhaps unaware of their options – were utilizing income-based repayment.[7]

For several years there was a push for the return of the 20/220 pathway, which calculated income versus loan burden and allowed deferment based on the resulting calculation; this permitted many residents, particularly those early in training, to defer their loans. This program was eliminated several years ago, however, and remains unavailable despite a number of organizations advocating for its return.

The "Pay as You Earn" program was proposed by President Obama in 2011. Similar to income-based plans, the program offered repayment based on a 15% to 10% decrease in monthly income. In addition, any debt remaining after 20 years would be forgiven. The plan was scheduled to officially take effect in 2014, but it has been available to select borrowers since 2012.[7] While the 20-year forgiveness is attractive, the reality is that a mere 10% of a physician's income will pay off most loans much sooner than that; this option may be most useful to borrowers with large families or financial hardships. There are several disadvantages to this program, however, including a higher overall interest charged over the life of the loan; additionally, while loans are forgiven after 20 years, taxes still apply.[2]

LOAN CONSOLIDATION

Consolidation is an option that allows a borrower to make one payment toward *all* loans instead of individual payments on *each* loan. This may simplify organization, but it does not change the interest rate, which reflects an average calculated from all the loans. Again, it is important to note that consolidation of pre-medical school loans or *early* consolidation of medical school loans may negate the six-month post-graduation grace period.

PUBLIC SERVICE LOAN FORGIVENESS PROGRAM

Employment in government-run or nonprofit organizations may allow loan forgiveness through the *Public Service Loan Forgiveness* program. Eligibility typically includes primary care work, such as family medicine or psychiatry, in an undeserved area for a delineated period of time. Two years of full-time service (30 hours a week) or four years of part-time service may provide a reward of up to $50,000. Certain public, federal, state or local government institutions also offer repayment forgiveness options for those surpassing 10 years of service, which require the borrower to pay only interest during that time period. These options typically are unavailable for those in emergency medicine, however, given emergency medicine's designation as a specialty; if working for a public institution, this option may be worth confirming.

STUDENT LOAN REFORMS

An initial attempt to relieve some of the financial burden of student loans occurred through the American Recovery and Reinvestment Act of 2009. $500 million in grant funding was given to the Health Resources and Service Administration, almost half of which went to those who worked in underserved areas. $300 million was given to the National Health Service Corps.[8] These changes have the greatest impact on *primary care specialties* and are unlikely to relieve the national burden of physician debt.

Through the Health Care and Education Reconciliation Act of 2010, public loans will be only available *directly* from the government, rather than through private lenders *backed* by the government (previously known as Federal Family Education Loans). This does not change private lending through banks without federal backing. The goal of this change is to prevent some of the extra charges incurred through bank loans, thereby decreasing interest rates and increasing maximum borrowing amounts.[9]

IMPACT ON SPECIALTY SELECTION

The increasing loan burden has had a major impact on medical students' decisions about which specialties to pursue; aware of the heavy financial implications, students are placing a much heavier weight on expected reimbursements. This means that lower-paid specialties, such as family and general internal medicine, are fast becoming less attractive career options. Choosing a more highly paid specialty has become a *necessity* for those carrying high debt loads. Primary care and preventative medicine, in particular, have taken strong hits.

Between 2000 and 2010, there was a 10% decrease in the number of active physicians in preventative medicine; this was mirrored by a similar decrease in first-year residents pursuing general medicine and family medicine between 2005 and 2010. This startling decline is in sharp contrast to the more than 10% *increase* in more lucrative specialties.[10]

With an ongoing shortage of primary care physicians, patient access to primary care has become problematic. In addition, many primary care physicians – in an attempt to relieve their own financial burdens – are refusing to see Medicaid and Medicare patients. This disparity often is bridged by emergency medicine, as *every* patient is afforded access to care in the ED. Patients without primary care providers and with no other options turn to the emergency department. Despite loan forgiveness programs designed to attract students to primary specialties, the shortage persists.

CONCLUSION

The cost of medical education continues to rise, adding to the skyrocketing debt burden of residents and young physicians. Resident physician salaries and loan repayment options fail to offer adequate solutions for eliminating this high volume of debt, leaving many new graduates financially overwhelmed. Although actions have been taken to relieve this national ailment, current policies have fallen short, leaving a trail of unintended consequences.

With the cost of medical school increasing at a rate twice that of inflation, it is estimated that 9% to 12% of after-tax income will be required to pay off loan debt in the decade following graduation.[9] The cost increase is a heavy burden for resident physicians and has become an influential factor in the migration of medical students to more lucrative specialties. Borrowers must be well-informed about the loans they receive and the repayment options available. In addition, borrowers must remain active in reducing the loan burden with unified petitions for change on both national and local levels. ✳

Additional Resources

- Loan Repayment options: http://studentaid.ed.gov/repay-loans/understand/plans
- Obama Memorandum: http://www.whitehouse.gov/the-press-office/2012/06/07/presidential-memorandum-improving-repayment-options-federal-student-loan

Chapter 15

PHYSICIAN SHORTAGES AND WORKFORCE ISSUES

Chadd K. Kraus, DO, MPH and Ellie Ventura, MD, MPH

The Council on Graduate Medical Education (COGME) predicts an increasing shortage of physicians in the coming years, speculating that by the year 2020 there will be a deficit of between 65,000 and 150,000 physicians.[1,2] A 2012 report released by the Association of American Medical Colleges confirms this unsettling reality; the United States is expected to experience a shortage of 124,000 full-time physicians by 2025, provided that physician supply and demand patterns remain unchanged.[2,5]

While the number of physicians in the workforce is expected to rise over the next 12 years, the U.S. population is predicted to grow by 50 million people (or 18%); the geriatric population is expected to increase from 35 million to 54 million. Overall growth – combined with an aging population and the rising prevalence of chronic diseases – quickly may outstrip the supply of doctors available to provide care, particularly in the emergency department.[3]

Approximately 20% of the U.S. population visits an ED each year.[4] The number of annual visits continues to grow, increasing from 94.9 million to 136.1 million between 1997 and 2011.[5,6] During the same period of time, hospital closures reduced the total number of EDs by 7%, placing an even greater demand on the emergency departments that remained.[5,6]

EMERGENCY MEDICINE RESIDENCY-TRAINED PHYSICIAN SHORTAGE

Physician shortages – which are compounded by physician lifestyle preferences, including shift work, decreasing call obligations, and work hour restrictions – impact emergency medicine in several ways. As of 2005, the supply of residency-trained emergency medicine specialists met only 58% of the required number of full-time equivalent physicians needed nationally.[7,8] Individual state percentages of emergency physician supply versus demand ranged from 10% in South Dakota to 104% in Hawaii.[7] Hawaii is the *only* state in the entire country with an adequate number of board-certified emergency physicians to fully staff its emergency departments;[7] Texas and Florida have the largest shortages in absolute numbers.[7]

A 2008 study estimated that, with constant growth and no attrition (including no deaths or disability) to reach saturation, it would take until 2019 to reverse the country's physician shortage.[2] Reasonable estimates of attrition based on research data indicate that approximately 450 emergency physicians leave the clinical workforce every year; however, 1,350 new physicians graduate from residency and replace those lost.[9] Even with a modest 1.7% attrition rate, it will take approximately 30 years to fill all slots with board-certified, residency-trained emergency physicians.[2,9] (Figure 1)

Figure 1. Looming Physician Shortages

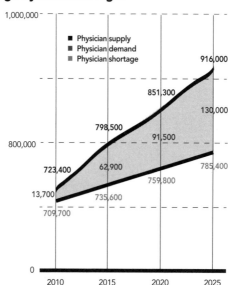

The Association of American Medical Colleges said national physician shortgages will be exacerbated by the expansion of coverage under the health system reform law and an aging population. The AAMC predicts a shortage of about 45,000 primary care physicians and 45,000 primary care physicians and 46,000 surgeons and medical specialists during the next decade. Above are projections for all physicians.

Adapted from the AAMC Center for Workforce Studies, June Analysis

According to an Institute of Medicine report, approximately 38% of practicing emergency department physicians are neither board-certified nor residency-trained in the specialty.[10,8] Smaller suburban and rural hospitals are particularly likely to be staffed by non-emergency medicine residency-trained physicians. Only 33% of physicians working in rural EDs are emergency medicine specialists; in comparison, 72% of those employed in urban areas are residency-trained or board-certified.[7,10] Most practitioners without an emergency medicine training background completed their residencies in family medicine or internal medicine.[8,10] Some rural EDs are staffed by midlevel providers alone.[7] The shortage in rural areas is expected to increase because so few new graduates of residency programs are willing to work in these areas.[7,8,10]

Of those emergency physicians who graduated within the past five years, only 5% are working in rural areas, compared to 15% of those who graduated at least 20 years ago.[8] Due to the ongoing shortage of board-certified and residency-trained emergency physicians, the utilization of non-residency trained physicians persists. The supply of emergency medicine-trained physicians, while growing, cannot meet short-term demand. Several studies have even suggested that supply will *never* meet demand under the current training and certification methods for emergency medicine physicians.[2,11] The insufficient number of emergency medicine specialists makes for disparate levels of training and experience, which may potentially affect clinical care.[11]

Even in areas where there *are* residency-trained emergency physicians, there exists shortages of other physicians who provide care emergency settings, including on-call consulting specialists. One survey of emergency department directors found that nearly 75% of EDs had problems related to a lack of on-call consultants[12] – an issue that also can hinder the adequacy of follow-up care for patients discharged home from the ED.[13]

PRIMARY CARE SHORTAGE

The shortage of primary care physicians adversely impacts patient care; the use of emergency departments may grow as a result of the widening gap between physician supply and demand. COGME's *Third Report* estimates that, ideally, *half* of the physician workforce would need to practice primary care medicine to effectively meet the medical needs of the country. This percentage is far greater than the 38% currently practicing primary care in the U.S. – an alarming statistic that also points to the declining number of medical school graduates choosing this path.[14]

The cause of this decline is multifactorial. Disparity in incomes between primary care and other specialties is of particular concern; reimbursement rates widely favor subspecialists over providers of primary care and preventive medicine. In addition, the traditional burden of a full panel of patients, the daunting component of practice-related business management, and on-call obligations seem onerous when compared to other specialties. Finally, some feel as though the traditional role of the primary care provider as the "provider of *all care*" has been eroded by the increased utilization of specialists.[15]

The Affordable Care Act will put new pressure on providers and payers to be more efficient and cost-effective as state and federal governments attempt to provide broader coverage while controlling costs. With the existing shortage of primary care physicians and decreasing reimbursements for these physicians, more patients may find their medical "homes" in the ED. Massachusetts introduced nearly universal insurance coverage in 2006, yet almost one-third of patients still report difficulty accessing care.[18] It is estimated that the additional 30 million insured individuals covered under the ACA will result in a shortage of nearly 20,000 additional physicians by the year 2020.[19] Much of the expansion of coverage under the ACA will occur through expansion of Medicaid. Because Medicaid patients historically have had relatively high rates of ED utilization, an increased demand for emergency care and emergency physicians is to be expected.[20,5]

UNEVEN DISTRIBUTION OF PROVIDERS

Physician shortages not only remain a function of the declining and insufficient number of providers; they also are a function of *geography*.

Density of physicians per 100,000 population[15,7]

Type	Large Urban	Large Rural	Small Rural
All	262	92.5	72
EM-trained and/or certified	10.3	5.3	2.5

According to the U.S. Census Bureau, 21% of our country's population lives in rural areas. Physicians are choosing to work in urban centers much more often than rural locations, leaving significant shortages of doctors outside our larger cities and creating a major health care obstacle for a large section of the population.[15]

The unequal geographic distribution of emergency physicians has been identified as one of the greatest challenges facing the emergency medicine workforce.[16] Only 12% of emergency physicians decide to seek employment in rural settings. One of the highest predictors of where residents will choose to practice upon graduation is the site of their graduate medical training[7,6]; most emergency medicine residency programs are located in urban areas.[6] RRC requirements make rural residency programs in emergency medicine nearly impossible to maintain, primarily due to lack of patient volume and acuity. There are other disincentives to rural practice, as well, including comparatively lower pay, longer work hours, and the requirement to provide more back-up call.[6,7,17]

SOLUTIONS

It will take more than one solution to the remedy the problem of physician shortages. Many options have been proposed, including the following:

Increase the yearly number of physicians in training. In 2012, U.S. medical schools saw a 3% increase in applications and a 1.5% increase in first-time enrollment.[23] Strong interest in medicine as a profession continues, as evidenced by increasing enrollment in U.S. medical schools. Fear of a future physician surplus, however, led to a recent cap on the number of Medicare-funded residency training positions.[24] This cap has been in place since 1997 without modification and is creating a challenge for new medical school graduates, who are competing for a limited number of residency positions.

The Affordable Care Act may relieve some of the bottleneck. The ACA allocated $1.5 billion for the National Health Services Corps from 2011 to 2015 to sponsor physicians willing to provide primary care in underserved areas.[21] It also reauthorizes funding for the expansion of residency programs through the Public Health Services Act.[21] Seventy-five percent of these positions are earmarked for primary care and general surgery, but a portion of the remainder may be allocated to emergency medicine.[22] One goal of the American College of Emergency Physician's 2010-2013 *Strategic Plan* is to ensure that a proportion of any newly created residency positions are designated for emergency medicine.[22]

Increase incentives for entering primary care. Although no single effort will improve primary care physician shortages, increases in the relative value units assigned by the Relative Value Scale Update Committee will improve reimbursement and may encourage future physicians to practice primary care. Revisions to the sustainable growth rate formula used to determine Medicare reimbursements – which adversely affect both primary care and emergency medicine – would help stabilize reimbursement and eliminate the agonizing choice that many physicians are forced to make when turning away Medicare patients based on unpredictable and potentially significant cuts in reimbursement.[25,26,27]

Optimize distribution of physicians. This goal can be achieved by supporting the continuation and growth of federal and state programs that incentivize rural medicine in return for medical school tuition assistance and student loan debt aid; such programs include the National Health Service Corps and the Community Health Center Program. Revisions to the *Health Professional Shortage Area* and *Medically Underserved Area/Population* criteria could help pinpoint areas in need.[28] ACEP and EMRA have been active in efforts to identify ways to provide loan repayment and other incentives to emergency medicine residency graduates willing to work in rural areas.[29]

The Institute of Medicine encourages rural hospitals to partner with academic health centers to enhance opportunities for professional consultations, telemedicine, patient referrals and continuing professional education.[9] Rural hospitals can benefit from emergency medicine residency-trained, board-certified physicians willing to offer education and support to ED providers who are trained in other specialties.[17,10] This assistance either could be provided by a physician on-site or at an academic medical center linked through telemedicine. Implementing these steps would help narrow the gap between urban and rural care, in light of continuing disparities in physician coverage. The use of ED providers and physicians not formally trained in emergency medicine remains controversial and is a topic of ongoing debate.

RESIDENCY TRAINING FOCUSED ON RURAL PRACTICE

Although many authors have accepted the common reality of non-physician providers and non-emergency medicine-trained physicians practicing in rural EDs, there are effective ways to recruit more residency-trained emergency physicians to these remote locations. For example, evidence shows that exposing residents to rural rotations during training increases resident selection of rural jobs;[30] these rural ED experiences are clinically similar to urban experiences.[31]

CONCLUSION

The entire U.S. health care system, including the specialty of emergency medicine, is facing a severe physician workforce shortage. Increasing physician education, creating incentives for areas in need, and redistributing existing physicians should be considered when addressing the growing problem. As recent graduates and passionate participants in the system, young physicians increasingly will become an important voice of change as these issues move forward. ✶

With thanks to George Leach, MD for his authorship of a previous version of this chapter.

Chapter ✦ 16 ✦

CHALLENGES OF SPECIALIST CARE

Sarah M. Schlein, MD

Access to consultant specialist physicians is a vital element of the care we provide in our emergency departments. Maintaining adequate consultant coverage is a multifactorial challenge that we must address to best serve our patients.

A 2010 national survey of medical directors found 74% of emergency departments experience a shortage of physicians willing to take emergency calls.[1] Specialty physician coverage is critical to the quality of care provided and the flow of patients in emergency departments. Over the last decade, consultant retention has become a growing issue of concern for emergency physicians.[2,3] By law, hospitals with Medicare funding are required to develop protocols for meeting the needs of patients requiring non-emergency medicine specialists.[4] Recent studies suggest that ED patients are now waiting longer for on-call specialist care and often have to be transferred significant distances to receive that care.[5] Multiple federal and state laws impact this issue and influence patient care, the etiology of this crisis, and its potential solutions (Table 1.)

EMTALA AND SPECIALIST OBLIGATIONS

Of the 98% of hospitals that depend on Medicare funding, all are required by federal statute to provide the same specialist care to hospital inpatients as they do to patients in their emergency departments.[6] Under EMTALA, any specialty practice with three or more specialist physicians initially was required to provide on-call, 24-hour coverage.[7]

> High acuity, the lack of previously established patient relationships, and an increased risk of negative outcomes make procedures performed on ED patients inherently riskier, leading to higher insurance premiums for physicians taking call.

A 2003 EMTALA revision, however, altered which hospitals are required to provide on-call coverage; the updated rule states that 24-hour coverage is *not required* for *underrepresented specialties* for which coverage provision is deemed "unfeasible."[8] This change has afforded hospitals greater flexibility in deciding if and when they provide this service. A clearly defined expectation no longer exists, and there is no minimum requirement for frequency of on-call coverage. Additional coverage standards can be further determined by individual hospital rules, hospital employee by-laws, or state regulations.

The most recent EMTALA revision offers hospitals the option of engaging in a *community call plan* (CCP) to share on-call responsibilities.[9] This permits non-emergency on-call specialists to have simultaneous on-call duties at multiple institutions and to schedule elective procedures, patient encounters, and surgeries while "on-call."[10] Specialty providers who refuse to take calls in their subspecialties may continue to treat only paying patients,[11] thus limiting the pool of specialists available for EMTALA-mandated care.

SPECIALIST RELUCTANCE TO TAKE CALLS

Emergency calls no longer are considered an absolute responsibility for all practicing physicians. Traditionally, on-call coverage was accepted as a required part of a physician's medical staff privileges and an opportunity to build one's practice. This professional standard has changed. Anecdotal reports indicate that non-emergency medicine specialists often have difficulty obtaining fair payment for emergency and trauma care due to high numbers of ED visits by uninsured and Medicaid patients.[12] With the implementation of the Affordable Care Act, the number of uninsured patients will decline, but there will continue to be an estimated 23 million uninsured Americans. This uninsured group includes all patients with incomes below the threshold to file taxes, prisoners, Native Americans, those living in the U.S. who are undocumented, and those who would incur premiums greater than 8% of their incomes.[13] All the above listed groups will continue to receive emergency care under EMTALA; thus the ACA will not eliminate the presence of uninsured patients in the ED.

Additionally, the ACA is expected to lead to increases in Medicaid patient visits. In 2010, 15% of Medicaid beneficiaries under age 65 averaged two or more emergency department visits in a 12-month period, making this group the patient population with the highest rate of ED visits.[14,15] There is a potential risk that increasing the percentage of Medicaid patients could further deter specialists' willingness to take calls; it also is unclear how reimbursement from this growing patient population will affect consultant motivation. Under the ACA, if a health insurance plan covers any emergency service, then it must also cover any out-of-network specialty care provided as part of the patient's care. Thus, specialists who contribute to an insured patient's care will receive payments that meet a minimum standard.[16]

Liability coverage also factors into a specialist's cost-benefit analysis. High acuity, the lack of previously established patient relationships, and an increased risk of negative outcomes make procedures performed on ED patients inherently riskier, leading to higher insurance premiums for physicians taking call. HR 36, recently introduced in the 113th Congress, could address this problem by improving the liability climate for emergency care. Under this legislation, emergency physicians and others providing care in EDs under EMTALA would be extended the same liability protections as public health service officers under the Federal Tort Claims Act.[17] It is important to note, however, that this bill has been introduced repeatedly since 2005 and has yet to pass in Congress.

These issues are further compounded by the current trend of placing increased importance on physician work-life balance. Under EMTALA, on-call physicians must be available to respond and physically come to the ED on short notice. The names of those that *fail* to respond, leading to patient transfer by requirement, are noted on the EMTALA transfer form. The receiving hospital has an obligation to report the consultant, who can be subject to civil fines of up to $50,000, potential malpractice liability, and possible exclusion from Medicare.[18] The allotted response time varies from state to state,[19] but there is no federally defined time. In Missouri, surgery consultants are given a 30-minute response time limit[20]; New Jersey requires response by telephone within 20 minutes, then a shared decision determines a fair in-person response time, with the ED physician decision governing. New Jersey also requires an in-person response to be less than 60 minutes for patients under the age of 18;[21] the ED clinical provider determines whether the responding on-call physician may send a resident or if the situation requires an in-person attending physician.[22] These requirements restrict living options and limit a physician from taking calls from home; this may conflict with the health care system's new focus on lifestyle and physician life balance.

Table 1. Laws Governing Consultants of Emergency Services

	Medicare	EMTALA	ACA	States
Current Law	Hospitals are required to provide the same specialist services to patients in the emergency department as they offer their non-ED patients.	Hospitals are required to maintain a list of on-call physicians for the ED.[34] On-call physicians must respond in a **reasonable** period of time. On-call specialists can receive a penalty of $50,000 if they do not present to the ED in a timely manner.[35]	All insurance plans that cover emergency services will be required to make a minimum payment to out-of-network on-call specialists who provide care associated with an ED visit.	Time for on-call physician response varies depending on state regulation. In most states, time to response is not addressed. Missouri: 30 minutes for surgery consultants.[36] New Jersey: 20 minutes for phone response ; <60 minute in-person response for patients <18 yrs;[37] ED provider can require attending in-person.[38]

INADEQUATE SPECIALTY WORKFORCE

By 2020, demand is expected to outstrip supply in multiple specialties, with non-primary care specialties experiencing a shortage of 46,100 to 62,400.[23] General surgery will see a shortage of 21,400; in fact, the number of practicing general surgeons is expected to fall from 39,100 (in the year 2000) to 30,800 by 2020. Ophthalmology and orthopedic surgery are each expected to need more than 6,000 additional physicians over current levels.[24]

One-third of practicing U.S. physicians are expected to retire in the next decade.[25] Rural surgeons are, on average, older than their urban counterparts; this trend is increasing.[26] There also has been an increase in the percentage of physicians who work more flexible schedules. In 2005, 7% of male physicians and 29% of female physicians worked part-time; by 2011, 22% of male and 44% of female doctors worked limited hours.[27] Given the aging U.S. population and the corresponding increase in need for surgical care, there will be an inadequate surgical workforce to meet these demands. Hospital or group practice bylaws often allow older surgeons to opt out of call coverage, only exacerbating the situation.[10] While the ACA is making efforts to increase the number of trainees and improve reimbursement in primary care and general surgery, these increases and incentives do not include specialists.[28,29]

EFFECT ON TRAUMA AND EMERGENCY CARE

Surgical coverage is a cornerstone of trauma level designation. Without adequate surgical specialty coverage, a hospital cannot maintain its trauma certification.[28] In 2010, 23% of emergency department directors noted a downgrade or suspension of their trauma level designations due to on-call specialty shortages.[29] Reports reveal that the proportion of under- and uninsured patients in the emergency department correlates to unmet consultant coverage needs. Shortages were found to be greater in non-teaching institutions, lower-level trauma centers, and EDs in the southern region of the U.S. In 2004, ACEP conducted a national-level study, which revealed that 29% of emergency department directors reported an unmet need for neurosurgery coverage, 26% for hand surgery, and 21% for orthopedic surgery.[30]

In 2002, in response to rising malpractice premiums, over 60 orthopedic surgeons with the University of Nevada withdrew their contracts, causing the state's *only* Level I trauma center to close for 11 days. Similar instances have been reported throughout the country of decreased trauma status due to loss of specialists.[31] Between 1990-2005, 339 of the 1,125 existing trauma centers closed;[32] this decline raises serious concerns about our emergency care system's ability to handle trauma.

The ACA may offer some respite from this current downward trend. In 2010, it allocated $224 million for emergency and trauma services. This money will be directed toward the regionalization of trauma centers, as well as *Trauma Care Center Grants*, which provide funds that enable trauma centers to maintain their core missions, compensate them for uncompensated care, and provide emergency awards to centers at risk of closure.[33] Other grants address shortfalls in trauma services and improve the availability of and access to these essential lifesaving services via state allocation. As of 2013, multiple federal and state programs impact the practice of emergency service consultants.

FUTURE CHALLENGES AND SOLUTIONS

Providing access to emergency and on-call services reflects how we prioritize the health of our public. At this time, however, individual physicians are not required to participate in order to meet the on-call mandates placed on hospitals. There remains a paucity of financial and other incentives for specialists and an unsolved liability problem. Even if system incentives were to be realigned, supply of potential on-call specialists is neither currently sufficient nor on a trajectory to meet projected demands.

Simple policies such as preferential operating room scheduling, meal coverage, or better parking may incentivize specialists and help hospitals improve their on-call coverage. The greatest gains, however, would come from making emergency care profitable enough that it becomes a competitive niche. Clearly, hospital requirements alone are insufficient to generate a complete on-call workforce. Such constraints can lead to poor retention of much-needed specialists.

Medicare and EMTALA regulations provide a framework, but an incentive-based system could provide a *real solution*. The ACA has taken steps to address several of the challenges related to retaining consultants. We also are seeing the emergence of *acute care surgery*, a model that limits specialists' responsibilities to emergent surgery or trauma. New on-call independent contracting groups, management companies, and hospitals that directly contract with specialists are possible market-driven solutions to improving coverage of on-call specialists in the health care system. For more than 20 years, California-based *EA Health* has been managing ED on-call compensation programs. Using a fee-for-service model, the provider, EA Health's administration, and the hospital divvy up earnings in a way that has ensured satisfaction for all parties. The on-call provider response times and decreased ED length of stay times have resulted in savings that offset the initial hospital costs.[39,40]

Unfortunately, EMTALA does not offer funding or liability coverage for on-call physicians, despite the legal mandate for specialist coverage. From a funding standpoint, the ACA now benefits *all* specialists; regardless of their patients' insurance network status, specialists will be reimbursed for the care they provide insured ED patients. This addresses neither the 30 million remaining *uninsured* patients, of course, nor the liability crisis. Efforts to promote legislation to improve liability coverage for physicians who partake in EMTALA-mandated care have yet to see success.[41]

There are multiple options for improving the available workforce. The medical training process, with limits on medical school and residency positions, is not on track to provide adequate access to physicians. Particularly in rural locations, the ACA's efforts to improve the number of primary care physicians could be extended to much-needed medical specialties to ensure adequate coverage for patients needing emergency care.

One potential way to improve coverage is through the use of midlevel providers for surgical services. Physician assistants (PAs) are a rapidly growing workforce that is projected to grow by 30% from 2010 to 2020.[42,43] PAs are becoming a key part of emergency specialty care; since 2011 PAs have been able to specialize in cardiovascular and thoracic surgery, emergency medicine, nephrology, orthopedic surgery and psychiatry. EMTALA does not permit physicians to avoid "first call" or inclusion on the hospital on-call list;[44] however, under EMTALA, midlevel providers may be appropriate responders to calls placed to on-call physicians.

The regionalization of on-call systems is another potential solution that has garnered financial support under the ACA.[45] Pinpointing those locations where on-call specialist pools would be most effective also warrants further study and evaluation. With the gaining popularity of telemedicine and improved technology, the pool of potential on-call physicians increases.

CONCLUSION

As emergency physicians, we will continue to care for a large percentage of our country's Medicaid and uninsured populations. The strained capacity of the surgical workforce will impact our ability to provide essential treatment and may require us to increase the number of patients we must transfer. Delays in definitive management raise grave concerns about increased mortality and morbidity in emergency patients. To prevent bad outcomes, we need to build policies that will improve the fragile on-call consultant system. ✶

With thanks to Mitesh B. Rao, MD, MHS for his authorship of a previous version of this chapter.

Chapter 17

CONTROVERSIES IN BOARD CERTIFICATION

Nathan Deal, MD and Donald E. Stader III, MD

Within the landscape of medical specialties, emergency medicine is a relative newcomer. Although emergency care existed long before, it wasn't until 1979 that emergency medicine was recognized as the 23rd medical specialty by the American Medical Association (AMA) and the American Board of Medical Specialties (ABMS). Since that time, the field of emergency medicine has continued to grow at an incredible pace. More than 150 emergency medicine residencies now exist across the nation,[1] and over 26,000 board-certified emergency physicians are practicing today.[2]

Within the United States, there exist two traditional certifying boards that provide board certification in emergency medicine: the American Board of Emergency Medicine (ABEM) and the American Board of Osteopathic Emergency Medicine (ABOEM). The Board of Certification in Emergency Medicine (BCEM), a component of the American Board of Physician Specialties (ABPS), is a new organization attempting to provide board certification; it distinguishes itself from other emergency medicine boards by offering an alternative track toward certification, which does not require residency training in emergency medicine. This track circumvents the now widely accepted model of emergency medicine residency training as a condition of board certification, an exception that has created substantial controversy within the emergency medicine community.

A BRIEF HISTORY OF ABMS AND ABEM

At the turn of the 20th century, interest in specialty training and certification was growing within the medical community. The beginnings of residencies and fellowships were materializing, and the first specialty examining boards were coming into existence. Between 1917 and 1932, specialty boards of ophthalmology, otolaryngology, obstetrics and gynecology, and dermatology were established. A pivotal moment came in the summer of 1933, when representatives from these specialty boards – along with delegates from the AMA, AAMC and the Federation of State Medical Boards (FSMB) – convened during an American Medical Association meeting.[3] The group acknowledged that additional specialty examining boards would form in the near future and that the process of specialty certification should be overseen by an advisory council. This council, the Advisory Board of Medical Specialties (ABMS), would be composed of members from each of the individual specialty boards and was later renamed the *American* Board of Medical Specialties.[4]

The journey toward a specialty board in emergency medicine began in earnest in the 1970s. The American College of Emergency Physicians (ACEP) and the University Association of Emergency Medicine (UAEM), a predecessor to the Society of Academic Emergency Medicine (SAEM), recognized a need for the development of emergency medicine training programs, as well as a means of certification. Because of their work, emergency medicine gained acceptance within the medical community. In 1976, the American Board of Emergency Medicine was created, and in 1979 the ABMS recognized emergency medicine as the 23rd medical specialty.

RESIDENCY TRAINING, PRACTICE TRACKS, AND BOARD ELIGIBILITY

ABMS currently requires residency training for board certification, but this was not always the case. With the creation of any new specialty board, it was common practice to allow non-residency-trained physicians to take the certifying examination if they had worked in the specialty for a sufficient amount of time. This pathway to certification, often referred to as a "practice track," allowed physicians who trained before the era of a specialty's residencies to obtain board certification. From 1979 to 1988, ABEM allowed both residency-trained and practice track physicians to obtain board certification in emergency medicine. In 1988, ABEM discontinued the practice track as a means of eligibility, in effect requiring all future diplomats to complete an accredited emergency medicine residency.[5]

Before any ABMS specialty board candidate is allowed to sit for the examination, that physician must meet the necessary criteria to be "board-eligible." In order to be board-eligible for the current ABEM exam, a physician must:

1. graduate from an approved medical school
2. complete an accredited residency in emergency medicine
3. in most cases, hold a valid medical license.

On January 1, 2015 ABEM will add further stipulations to the term "board-eligible," the most significant of these being new time criteria. ABEM will allow a physician to remain board-eligible for a maximum of 10 years following residency graduation as long as the candidate continues to meet certain conditions, including the completion of continuing medical education.

THE DANIEL CASE

After the closure of the practice track toward ABEM certification, there remained a number of practicing emergency physicians who had not received board certification and who had not completed an emergency medicine residency. In 1990, Gregory Daniel, MD, and a collection of other plaintiffs sued ABEM to reopen the practice track to board certification. Many of these plaintiffs eventually established the Association of Disenfranchised Emergency Physicians, later renamed the Association of Emergency Physicians (AEP). The legal battle that ensued would last 15 years; in 2005, the Second Circuit Court of Appeals upheld a decision and dismissed all claims against ABEM.[6]

This legal decision legitimizes the long-held belief of many physicians that residency training is a necessary component in the education of a proficient physician. At present time, ABEM and all other specialty boards of ABMS continue to require residency training for certification eligibility. The controversy of board certification continues, however, with a number of physicians interested in searching out alternative means of board certification.

THE CREATION OF ABPS AND THE CONTROVERSY

The American Board of Physician Specialties (ABPS) exists as a competing organization to the ABMS. ABPS was created in 2005 as the parent organization to several specialty boards, including the Board of Certification in Emergency Medicine (BCEM), a direct competitor to ABEM.[7] The creation of these alternative boards has opened a separate gateway for emergency physicians who may not meet the requirements for ABEM board certification.

Controversy has surrounded the creation of BCEM, which allows non-emergency medicine residency-trained physicians to obtain board certification in the specialty. Currently the BCEM boasts three different requirement tracts that make a candidate eligible to sit for its exam. Two of these tracts offer eligibility after the candidate has completed a non-emergency medicine residency program and has worked in an emergency medicine setting for a required amount of time.

A collection of emergency medicine organizations, including EMRA, ACEP, and AAEM, have opposed the ABPS alternative board for a host of reasons. The central issue in the debate revolves around the necessity of emergency medicine residency training for board eligibility. EMRA has taken a firm stance against this channel and adamantly asserts that residency training in the specialty is a critical component in the training of a new emergency physician; EMRA also holds that residency training is the *sole* path to board certification. With the growing information and skillset required to be a competent emergency physician, residency training in the specialty is the superior route for emergency physicians and the patients they serve.

BOARD CERTIFICATION AND ADVERTISING

Regardless of which certifying board a physician chooses, it ultimately is up to individual state medical boards to determine whether a physician can be publicly advertised as "board-certified." Most states' medical boards strictly regulate the use of this term, having decided that declaring board certification may impact the decisions that patients make regarding their medical care. Until recently, the use of the term meant that the physician was certified by the ABMS, or possibly the AOA. Debate surrounds whether physicians who are certified by BCEM should be permitted to advertise themselves in an equivalent manner to those who are certified through the ABMS.

FLORIDA, TEXAS AND THE SECOND CIRCUIT COURT

No federal legislation exists regarding board certification for physicians. Each state has the freedom to determine the criteria that must be meet, resulting in a patchwork of regulation. Over the past few years, ABPS and BCEM have asked for their processes to be considered equivalent to ABEM or AOBEM certification, which has resulted in several rulings by state medical boards and appeals courts regarding the status of board certification.

The first ruling came from the Florida Board of Medicine in 2001. At that time, the Florida board recognized BCEM certification as equal to that provided by ABMS or the AOA. Following the ruling, a collection of organizations, including EMRA, ACEP, the Florida College of Emergency Medicine, AAEM, and the Florida Medical Association, appealed to the board – without success – to reverse its decision. Currently, BCEM-certified physicians can continue to advertise themselves as "board certified" in Florida.[8]

The most recent challenge to board certification came from Texas. Beginning in 2009, ABPS asked the Texas Medical Board (TMB) if the language being used would recognize ABPS as an equivalent certifying body. Without full evaluation, TMB issued a response suggesting that BCEM-certified physicians were, indeed, permitted to advertise themselves as such. This decision prompted roughly 175 BCEM-certified physicians to begin advertising within Texas. Word quickly spread – and, again, EMRA, ACEP, the Texas College of Emergency Physicians, and a collection of partner organizations appealed to the TMB to fully evaluate the issue and clarify the regulatory language. In the fall of 2010, the TMB ruled that the BCEM-certified physicians who had been advertising themselves as board-certified could continue to do so; however, all *future* physicians who wish to advertise must complete a specialty-specific residency in order to meet the requirements of certification.

While state medical boards have been the stage for most certification battles, some of these issues have spilled over into the courts. The New York State Department of Health determined that BCEM certification was *not* equivalent to certification by ABMS or AOA; thus, BCEM physicians could not advertise themselves as board-certified. This resulted in a legal suit between the ABPS and the state's department of health, originally filed in 2006. In 2009, a district court ruled in New York's favor, citing the lack of specialty-specific training as an indication of the certifying bodies' inequity. This decision was appealed; in 2010, the second court of appeals affirmed the department of health's decision.[9]

CONCLUSION

Emergency medicine training and certification have developed rapidly since the recognition of the field in 1979; today, it is a widely accepted and influential specialty within the house of medicine. The term "board-certified" in emergency medicine has evolved over the past 30 years and now faces new challenges, as ABPS and BCEM attempt to provide alternative paths to certification. While several state medical boards have ruled on this issue – some allowing for equivalent advertising, and some opposing it – the fight will continue on a state by state basis. Advocates of BCEM and ABPS continue to appeal for parallel status. EMRA, ACEP and partner organizations will continue to defend what it means to be board-certified and to protect the public against those without sufficient training. EMRA holds the central belief that emergency medicine residency training is necessary to ensure the continued integrity of our specialty. It is important for emergency physicians, and especially those currently in training, to appeal to their state medical boards by advocating the importance of residency training and the need for truth in advertising with the use of the term "board-certified." ✶

Osteopathic Recognition and Training

The American Osteopathic Board of Emergency Physicians (AOBEM) offers eligibility for board certification for doctors of osteopathy (DOs) who have completed an American Osteopathic Association-approved residency in emergency medicine and who have either practiced for one year or have completed a year of subspecialty training. As of December 2011, a total of 2,152 emergency physicians were board-certified by AOBEM.[10] To meet this requirement, graduates of an American Osteopathic Association (AOA) emergency medicine program must pass an oral and a clinical examination.

In 2012, the ACGME took controversial steps to limit access to its fellowships by allowing eligibility only for graduates of ACGME residencies. This change prevents AOA residency graduates from participating in ACGME-accredited fellowships. This change has been strongly opposed by EMRA, ACEP, the Emergency Medicine RRC and other organizations in emergency medicine, which view AOA and ACGME residency programs as equivalent training. At the time of this publication, the ACGME was still deliberating on whether AOA residency-trained physicians would be eligible for ACGME-accredited fellowships.

Chapter 18

NON-PHYSICIAN PROVIDERS IN THE EMERGENCY DEPARTMENT

Robert Redwood, MD and Cameron A. Decker, MD

INTRODUCTION

The value of emergency medicine residency training and the role of physician leadership in emergency departments is under pressure from multiple sources. An increasing demand for services, an insufficient work force, duty hour restrictions, and various other factors have resulted in a growing number of non-physician providers seeking to offer care in the emergency department. While residency-trained, board-certified emergency physicians ideally would staff all EDs, health care market forces may no longer allow for the *gold standard*: "In fact, it is likely that [emergency physicians] will not be able to fill the workforce demand for several decades, if ever."[1]

This chapter addresses those providers with alternative educational backgrounds — outside of MD or DO — who seek to extend their scopes of practice into the roles traditionally filled by emergency physicians. The leading examples of non-physician providers (NPPs) beginning to practice alongside, and sometimes independently of, emergency physicians in emergency departments are physician assistants (PAs) and nurse practitioners (NPs).

While there is a valid argument that the practice doctorate can expand the workforce of accountable health care providers by creating additional clinical leaders and teachers, it must be weighed against the potential risks to patient safety and the inherent confusion of having multiple types of "doctors" with vastly different levels of training.

PHYSICIAN ASSISTANTS

A physician assistant is a health care provider who practices medicine under the supervision of a licensed physician. Most PA programs are master-level. Physician assistant education is based on the medical model and is designed to complement physician training; many PA programs are located in existing medical colleges and universities. The average training program is 26 to 27 months in duration without required specialty-specific instruction,[2,3] although a growing national trend toward post-graduate subspecialization — especially in emergency medicine — is well underway. State medical boards regulate professional licensure, and all states mandate that PA graduates pass a certifying examination administered by the National Commission on the Certification of Physician Assistants (NCCPA). The recertification exam is taken on a six-year cycle with a transition to extend to ten years. PAs must log 100 hours of continuing medical education every two years to maintain active certification. They exercise autonomy in patient care as determined by their supervising physicians, hospital policies, and state laws; however, they may not practice independently.

Of the more than 83,000 practicing physician assistants, 10.7% practice in emergency medicine, the second largest single PA specialty outside of primary care.[4] The overwhelming majority of emergency medicine PA training is obtained while on the job and through specialty-specific continuing education; only 10.68% of emergency medicine PAs pursue a one- to two-year post-graduate "fellowship" certification.[5] Currently, there are 19 emergency medicine PA residency programs in the United States; while the curriculum has not yet been standardized, the NCCPA has outlined a core competency model that likely will serve as the foundation for a future nationwide standardized curriculum.[6] The six core competencies, identical to those of the ACGME, are *medical knowledge, interpersonal and communication skills, patient care, professionalism, practiced-based learning and improvement,* and *systems-based practice.*

Emergency medicine PAs typically work rotations similar to those of emergency medicine resident physicians, although their weekly duty hours tend to be shorter and their patient acuity lower; they also are required to attend PA-specific didactic sessions. In lieu of a match process, PAs are required to complete a residency application, which is similar to a competitive job application and generally requires a letter of intent, an academic transcript, NCCPA board scores (if certified), a curriculum vitae, and letters of recommendation.

PAs may demonstrate mastery-level competence in the field by obtaining a *Certificate of Added Qualifications* (CAQ) in emergency medicine by the NCCPA. First offered in 2011, the CAQ requires 18 months of emergency medicine experience (3,000 hours), 150 hours of continuing education in the field, physician attestation of demonstrated procedural competencies, and completion of a certifying exam.[7] It is important to note that the CAQ is not an educational program, but a method of displaying proficiency.

NURSE PRACTITIONERS

Nurse practitioners are registered nurses with additional specific advanced nursing education, typically a master's-level degree. Unlike the medical model applied in physician assistant training, which emphasizes treatment of disease processes, NP training applies a nursing model to education that emphasizes *how* to care for the patient. As one program explains, the nursing model is *biopsychosocial-centered,* emphasizing disease adaptation, health promotion, wellness, and prevention.[8] Like

PAs, NPs are licensed at the state level, although typically through nursing boards rather than medical boards. The American Academy of Nurse Practitioners (AANP) and the American Nurses Credentialing Center (ANCC) are two credentialing bodies that offer certifications in nursing; these certifications must be renewed every five years in order to continue development within the profession. While generally considered "midlevel" providers, NPs – unlike PAs – may be licensed to practice independently of direct physician supervision in some states.

During an NP master's degree or emergency nurse practitioner (ENP) fellowship, the training emphasizes a blend of clinical and academic training and can be pursued full-time or part-time (often while the participant works as a registered nurse). A typical program requires between 36 and 54 classroom credits and 700 to 1,500 clinical hours. Admission requirements vary, but an NP applicant typically must hold a bachelor's degree, must have more than 700 hours of clinical nursing experience, and must have earned a passing score on the National Council Licensure Examination.

While a PA may enter his or her formal training with virtually any level of health care experience, most NP students have significant prior nursing experience. An NP is a registered nurse who "has acquired the expert knowledge base, complex decision-making skills, and clinical competencies for expanded practice."[9] The nine core competencies of the NP are *scientific foundation, leadership, quality, practice inquiry, technology and information literacy, policy, health delivery systems, ethics,* and *independent practice.*[10] In the National Organization of Nurse Practitioner Faculties' policy statement on the core competencies, the independent practice section specifically notes that an NP should function as "a licensed independent practitioner...independently manage diagnosed and undiagnosed patients...[and] prescribe medications within the scope of practice."[11]

The emergency nurse practitioner fellowship is a specialized NP degree that requires a similar time commitment to that required by family health or acute care NP degrees. The ENP is an uncommon niche in the United States, and most NPs desiring to work in acute care settings elect to pursue family health NPs and then apply directly for ED or urgent care positions. There are six ENP fellowships offered in the U.S. Although there is no national standardized curriculum for the ENP fellowship, the program at Emory University offers a representative curriculum that includes "basic and advanced suturing, joint injection, slit lamp examinations, and splinting and casting. Students are given more than 700 clock-hours of supervised clinical experiences in areas such as women's health, pediatrics, family practice, fast track non-acute emergency settings, and high-acuity emergency settings."[12] While designated as an ENP fellow, the practitioner sits for the Family Nurse Practitioner (FNP) exam at the conclusion of training. The Acute Care Nurse Practitioner program is not often selected by candidates who wish to work in an ED setting, as it is limited to adult care.

ROLE OF NON-PHYSICIAN PRACTITIONERS IN EMERGENCY MEDICINE

According to a recent emergency physician workforce study, the approximately 22,000 board-certified emergency physicians falls drastically short of the 40,030 needed to staff all 4,828 EDs in the United States (55% of demand met). By these estimates, the unrealistic "best-case/no-attrition scenario" would result in all EDs being staffed with board-certified emergency physicians by 2019. A more reasonable intermediate scenario (2.5% attrition) would satisfy workforce needs by 2038.[13] Compounding the situation, the recent economic recession saw employer-based health care coverage drop from 60.4 % to 55.9% from 2007 to 2009, a problem that may add additional patient visits to already overcrowded EDs.[14]

How to address this workforce shortage is an ongoing debate, but most agree that NPPs will be an essential component of the long-term solution. Researchers note that "physician supply shortages in all fields contribute to — and will continue to contribute to — a situation where providers with other levels of training may be a necessary part of the workforce for the foreseeable future."[15]

In 2006, NPPs provided care for greater than 12% of ED patients; over half of these patients were also seen by a staff physician. Further, more than 77% of EDs reported the use of an NPP.[16] The U.S. General Accounting Office estimates that the NPP workforce across all specialties "includes 79,980 PAs, with 93% in clinical practice [as well as] 141,209 NPs in the United States, of whom 85% are in primary care. Only 5% of NPPs practice in emergency care settings."[17] The typical emergency medicine PA practice model is that of "physician extension," where a PA independently sees low-acuity patients with on-site physician back-up.

The physician is consulted if the case becomes more complicated or if the PA has questions about diagnosis or management. In fact, 74.45% of emergency medicine PAs solely work under the direction of an on-site attending, and only 5.93% report working strictly with off-site supervision.[18] On the other hand, ENPs and FNPs often work independently in urgent care centers and small community emergency departments. The latter arrangement is essentially contradictory to Schneider, et al.'s observation: "physician assistants and nurse practitioners can be used to augment emergency physicians, but in small departments, which represent a sizable percentage of facilities, solo coverage by a physician may still be preferable."[19]

While different provider groups inevitably will have a wide range of opinions on the ideal staffing of our nation's EDs, the reality is that cost-effective care and appropriate stewardship of scarce resources will have a significant impact on the blend of emergency physicians and NPPs meeting the ever-expanding coverage needs. In terms of cost versus productivity, the average PA (across all specialties) earns $94,870 annually and sees 80.47 patients per week.[20] The average NP (across all specialties) earns $90,583 annually and typically sees 64.95 patients per week.[21] Comparing these figures to emergency physicians, who earn $237,000 annually and see an average 92 patients per week,[22] NPPs may offer a significant cost savings by treating low-acuity patients, freeing physicians to focus on those with higher acuity. When analyzing cost effectiveness, however, one must also take into account physician-specific administrative and educational duties, such as providing EMS medical direction and overseeing learners, including NPPs, residents, and medical students.

PUSH FOR EXPANSION

The push for expansion among NPPs can be broken down into two separate initiatives. The first is a movement to expand the duties and competencies of NPPs into advanced procedures and therapies typically performed by emergency physicians; the other is to expand their autonomy, which would allow NPPs to work independent of physician oversight. These initiatives are highly contested among NPP professional groups and physician groups alike and will undoubtedly shape the future of the health care workforce. The expansion of NPP roles already has become a prominent discussion point in the allocation of training funds under the Affordable Care Act (ACA).[23] Regardless of emergency medicine training and accreditation, the objective of every emergency physician and NPP is to provide safe, effective patient care; a thoughtful discussion about the appropriate roles of emergency providers is crucial to achieving this shared goal.

EXPANDED DUTIES

A 2005 study reports that, of all patients cared for by NPPs, approximately 6% arrive by ambulance, 37% have urgent or emergent acuity, and 3% are admitted. Although the acuity data is lower than in patients seen by emergency physicians, the message is clear that "the role of midlevel providers, who may practice without on-site physician involvement, has clearly extended beyond minor presentations."[24] It should be noted that this phenomenon appears to be more specific to physician assistants; the role of PAs in busier urban EDs continues to outpace that of nurse practitioners, who tend to staff more urgent care clinics and rural emergency departments.

The claim that NPP scope of practice has crept into the critical care patient population traditionally managed by physicians is bolstered by a recent nationwide survey of more than 5,000 emergency medicine PAs; 43.1% reported performing rapid sequence intubation; 35.9%, central venous access; 34.7%, tube thoracostomies; and 54.0%, procedural sedation.[25] While some physicians view this expansion as a welcome – if incomplete – solution to the ever-widening patient-to-provider ratio, others have voiced concerns regarding patient safety. Is there a discrepancy between the "top" of an NPP's *license* and the "top" of his or her *expertise*? Limited data address the quality and safety of NPPs caring for higher acuity ED patients; however, a recent study of 4,029 visits for acute asthma in 63 U.S. emergency departments found that unsupervised NPPs provided a lower quality of ED asthma care than physician-supervised NPPs and physicians alone.[26]

Of the two debates, the trend of NPPs (specifically PAs) seeing higher acuity patients is probably less controversial among emergency physicians than the debate over the push for *autonomy*, as most of this expansion has taken place under appropriate physician supervision. Provided that patient care is not compromised, NPPs seeing higher acuity patients may allow physicians to be more efficient, focus on the most critically ill patients; patient satisfaction also may improve through decreased wait times and more personal interaction with their providers. That being said, the current EMRA Council resolution on the matter clearly states: "Due to the extensive fund of knowledge, skill set, and training required for delivery of appropriate, competent emergency care, the role of [NPPs] in the [ED] should remain limited to that of fast track or non-acute care settings with continued oversight by an [EP]."[27] Given the dynamic landscape of emergency medicine, NPP policy and practice will continue to evolve.

EXPANDED AUTONOMY

The push for autonomy by some members of the NPP community is extremely controversial among emergency physicians and raises concerns regarding patient safety, dilution of the "midlevel provider" workforce, and confusion among patients regarding their provider's level of training and expertise. This movement toward expansion is motivated not just by the NPPs themselves, but also by the needs of the health care system as a whole. In general, proponents of the movement desire NPPs to be able to practice independently with little or no physician oversight. Some researchers have taken a clear stance on the issue, asserting "the onus will be on emergency physicians and their professional societies to provide [NPPs] with adequate supervision when needed and more widely available educational opportunities."[28]

The American Academy of Emergency Medicine has taken an even firmer stance, issuing a policy statement affirming that "patients [should] have timely access to the most appropriate and qualified practitioners. A physician assistant/nurse practitioner is an assistant and should never be utilized to replace a physician. Attending physicians must be physically present, accessible, and be permitted adequate time to be directly involved in supervision of care."[29] The American College of Emergency Physicians echoes this belief in a 2007 policy statement: "PAs and NPs may be placed in clinical and administrative situations in which they will supplement and assist emergency physicians. PAs and NPs do not replace the medical expertise and patient care provided by emergency physicians."[30]

The issue of patient safety undoubtedly will become the central focus of this debate as quality measures begin to play an increasingly important role in the health care system, including payments to hospitals and providers. Unfortunately, literature on the quality of care provided by NPPs remains sparse. Interestingly, the bulk of research on NPP outcomes in the ED has focused on quality measures apart from treatment outcomes. For example, four Canadian reviews report the results of primary studies regarding the effect of NPPs on ED system outcomes. These studies showed an improvement in achieving wait-time benchmarks for patients visiting the ED after NPP implementation, as well as a 9% shorter length of stay.[31]

Regarding specific value-added benefits of a NPP workforce, a U.S survey of 290 emergency physicians who had worked with NPPs rated their performance highest in patient education, history, and physical examination; and slightly lower in diagnosis and clinical management. Respondents also rated NPPs' overall utility, cost-effectiveness and capability in the ED at 5.0 to 5.4 on a seven-point scale, but felt that the general training of NPPs did not provide enough emergency medicine education.[32] Ultimately, this debate will continue until large, multicenter studies are published, comparing clinical outcomes of emergency physicians and NPPs.

A second concern has been proposed regarding advanced training requirements and independent NPPs: the advanced training diminishes the returns of a standard PA or NP role, putting a further stress on our already overworked midlevel provider workforce. Additional education mandates for PAs and NPs may, in fact, deter those who would pursue such careers due to the increasing financial investment and time commitment.[33] If the practice doctorate or subspecialized PA siphons from the pool of available nurses and general PAs, the provider shortage could presumably worsen. Along these lines, the practice doctorate and subspecialized PA could compound existing staffing issues and compromise the ACA's ability to expand access to care.

Some also question the level of expertise and training quality of NPPs. While a master's level NP or PA degree equates to roughly 1,000-1,500 clinical hours, the clinical *years* of medical school and residency equate to 14,000-15,000 clinical hours.[34] The practice doctorate degree is not yet standardized nationwide, but it generally adds an additional 1,000-2,000 clinical hours above the nurse practitioner degree, with specific emphasis on leadership, interpretation of evidence-based medicine, and health policy. The American Association of Colleges of Nursing (AACN) has expressed interest in phasing out NP programs altogether and transitioning all advanced practice nursing education to the level of practice doctorate degree by 2015.[35] Many nursing professionals with this doctorate degree feel that their educational backgrounds should permit them to introduce themselves to patients *as doctors*.

While there is a valid argument that the practice doctorate can expand the workforce of accountable health care providers by creating additional clinical leaders and teachers, it must be weighed against the potential risks to patient safety and the inherent confusion of having multiple types of "doctors" with vastly different levels of training. Contradicting the notion that – under our current trajectory – "traditional titles like physician and nurse will blur as we transcend disciplines and overlapping roles,"[36] The American Medical Association passed Resolution 211, which aims to eliminate misrepresentation by schools or practitioners who claim that their education level is equivalent to that of a physician.[37]

CONCLUSION

Non-physician providers play a critical role in the emergency care infrastructure, especially in light of escalating workforce demands and the increasing number of ED visits. Emergency medicine is a team effort, however, that should be supervised by those individuals with the highest intensity of training: emergency physicians. The increased independence and expanded scope of practice of NPPs is a question of patient safety; it has obscured differences in qualifications for patients and at times has created a less collaborative approach to care. Leading scholars have expressed concerns that the rapid expansion of the NPP role in acute care settings has not been well-planned; their views should give us pause to consider this transition. EMRA holds that there are the distinct attributes and values unique to the emergency medicine residency-trained, board-certified physician's medical education. Regardless of our different opinions regarding degrees or independence of practice, we must work with our colleagues in other professions to build a better and safer future for our patients. ✴

With thanks to Taylor R. Spencer, MD, MPH for his authorship of a previous version of this chapter.

Chapter 19

ADVOCACY 101: GETTING INVOLVED

Michael M. Khouli, MD and Lindsay Harmon-Hardin, MD

> *"Medicine is a social science, and politics is nothing else but medicine on a large scale."* — Rudolf Virchow

As emergency medicine physicians, we are constantly confronted with individual patients suffering the medical consequences of broader social and environmental factors and the effects of health policy. While routinely advocating for our patients' immediate health care needs to nurses, consultants, and administrators, residents often feel passionate about addressing those social circumstances that contribute to the underlying burden of disease. Beyond the role of bedside physician, they wish to be community advocates, but may feel overwhelmed by constraints on their time and daunted by the complexities of the political process. Legislators, with the scores of people and organizations competing for their attention, may seem an unfamiliar and inaccessible audience. Despite recent calls for innovation, traditional residency curricula have offered little formal training in political and community advocacy.[1-3]

As advocacy becomes increasingly integral to the medical profession, physicians need to be recognized for their expertise, and their advocacy efforts need to be acknowledged for what they are – true scholarly pursuits.

WHY ADVOCATE?

According to the ACEP code of ethics, emergency physicians have an ethical duty to promote population health through advocacy, participating "in efforts to educate others about the potential of well-designed laws, programs, and policies to improve the overall health and safety of the public."[4] Physician advocacy can range from working toward state health care reform to advising a local school board.[3] Advocacy activities might include attending a physicians' day at the state house, testifying before a committee, or corresponding and meeting one-on-one with an elected official.[5]

It may seem unlikely that a letter or conversation from an individual physician could impact public policy, but multiple cases demonstrate that physicians *can*, indeed, affect legislation. Two physicians working with the Canadian Association of Emergency Physicians, for example, influenced the government to enact one of the most stringent gun regulations in the Western Hemisphere, contributing to a 37% drop in gun-related deaths in the years following the law's enactment.[6,7] As our nation continues the process of health care reform, effective physician advocacy is more important than ever.

FINDING YOUR PASSION

Various authors have outlined different frameworks for physician advocacy, but in the words of Canadian physician, Jatina Lai, MD, "Advocacy is optimized when it arises from a foundation of passion."[6,8,9] As emergency physicians, we are confronted during virtually every shift with things we wish we could change; determine what you care about, and you will find your advocacy goal. This sounds simple and often is. The EMRA and ACEP websites feature discussions on many issues that may address your specific concerns. Given our perspective from the frontlines of health care, emergency physicians are uniquely positioned to identify broad health problems. The ED truly is a "room with a view,"[10] which affords us ample opportunity to translate our passion to advocacy.

BE INFORMED

Research your topic thoroughly and know your subject matter. Moreover, understand your opponents' arguments, which will enable you to preempt criticism of your position in advance of any meetings with policymakers. If you are advocating for stricter gun control, for example, you may want to peruse the National Rifle Association website. If you are dealing with a state issue, research when and how other states have addressed it; be familiar with current legislation on your topic and understand you legislator's perspective. What committees is she on and what does her prior voting record show? What are her key constituencies? Congressional websites contain extensive information about the personal and professional background of legislators.

ADVOCACY AS LEADERSHIP

While it is crucial to demonstrate a detailed understanding of your issue, remember that you already are well-positioned to make an impact. Your role as a physician gives you a great deal of clout; physicians enjoy considerable social status and respect as healers, scholars, and public servants. A survey of legislative assistants reported that 90% of physician lobbyists were either *very effective* or *somewhat effective* – and, in the words of one legislative assistant, "should recognize the power they have to influence Congress."[11] Moreover, within the current health care system, emergency physicians provide a disproportionate share of the care for the underinsured – far more than any other medical specialists.[12] This further sets our specialty apart and gives us a more powerful voice in the public policy debate.

Partnering with supportive organizations such as EMRA, ACEP, AMA, or a local grassroots network can add strength in numbers to your issue, making legislators more likely to respond and act. Additionally, these professional organizations already may have researched and laid the groundwork needed to present your issue; their government affairs staff may have established relationships with legislators and can help refine and tailor your arguments.[13] They may offer contacts to like-minded interest groups and lobbyists who wish to be involved and will eventually be included in the policymaking process. Inviting such groups to the discussion early can earn valuable allies, bolster support, and facilitate passage of a bill. Just as modern medical paradigms incorporate a health care team with a physician as team leader, advocacy is strengthened by various members bringing diverse knowledge and skills to the table.[9]

ESTABLISH CONTACT

You may reach out to a legislator much like you would contact another physician about a patient in the emergency department. First, identify yourself and whether you are a constituent. Do not be surprised if you are asked to provide a specific home or work address; legislators tend to give more heed to constituents from their own districts. After providing your personal information, immediately state the issue you would like to address. Next, tell your story and supply supporting evidence. Be clear, concise, and organized; avoid medical terminology. Finally, explicitly state your request. You may want your legislator to introduce, support, or oppose specific legislation; introduce an amendment to an existing bill; or talk to other legislators about an issue.

Personal stories are more influential than reams of statistics or references. Statistics often will be ignored; stories, which are more memorable and are processed better by the human brain, generate greater sympathy than numerical statistics.[15] A personal story can give a "face" to an issue and help legislators contextualize and connect with the patient or situation. Well-placed statistics can be used to support your story, but they should be kept to a minimum. Again, be concise and focused; less is more. Using your prior knowledge of the legislator's background, seek to frame the issue from his or her standpoint, rather than explaining why it matters to *you*. Finally, you may offer to have the legislator visit your emergency department, where a greater insight into your concerns can be gained.[16]

Finding Your Legislators

Start by determining which level of government (local, state, or federal) has jurisdiction over your issue; in some cases, it may be both state and federal. Some programs, such as Medicaid, are shared between jurisdictions.[14] Once you know which area of government to target, identify your particular legislators. The following websites will aid you in finding the pertinent contact information:

> *www.house.gov*
> *www.senate.gov*
> *www.acep.org (Advocacy section)*
> *www.votesmart.com*

Snail Mail

While traditional mail largely has been supplanted by electronic communication, letters sent via the postal service remain highly effective. A tangible letter stands out more than one among dozens of daily emails and demonstrates that you did more than just cut and paste. Use a standard format; a single page should be sufficient, summarizing one or two key issues in language an educated layperson can understand.[13] The following is one example.

Jane W. Doe, MD
500 West Way
Indianapolis, IN 40000

January 1, 2013

The Honorable P. Smith
Indiana Senate
Indianapolis, IN 40000

Dear Senator Smith,

I am a constituent of yours from Franklin County, writing to ask for your support of the proposed bicycle helmet law (Senate Bill 400). As an emergency medicine physician, I see many children present to the emergency department with head injuries that could have been prevented by wearing a bicycle helmet. The story of Billy K., also from Franklin County, stands out in my mind. He is a five-year-old who was just learning to ride his bike. No one on his street or in his family had ever worn a bicycle helmet; they were not even aware it was a safety concern. When Billy arrived to the emergency department, he was confused and had a large cut overlying a skull fracture to the back of his head. After a week in the hospital Billy went home, but had he worn a helmet, he might not have been injured at all. Fortunately, he was able to return to normal activities, but not all children are so lucky. Approximately 7% of all brain injuries are related to bicycle accidents;[17] one study shows that the use of bicycle helmets can reduce the risk of head injury by 74 to 85%.[18] Finally, the CDC recommends that states increase helmet use by implementing legislation, education, and enforcement. If you have any questions about my personal experience or the research regarding bicycle helmet safety, please do not hesitate to contact me. Thank you for considering supporting Senate Bill 400.

Sincerely,
Jane W. Doe, MD

Email

The ease and speed of email have made it a convenient way for the public to contact legislators; however, this ease and convenience can discredit its content. Mass template emails asking citizens to add their names before forwarding them to representatives are tallied and then promptly dismissed by legislative staff. To stand out, your email must demonstrate the same interest and passion as any other communication. The subject line of the email should state that you are a constituent and explain where you are from.[14] Draft your email as you would write a letter; include an *introduction, specific request, story, supporting statistics, repeated request*, and a *thank you*. Personalization will improve the chances of your email being read and considered by the legislator.

Telephone

Like physicians, legislators are very busy. Taking the time to call legislative offices – in Washington D.C., in state, or locally – can be productive, but getting the opportunity to speak with a legislator is rare. More often, you will be directed to a legislative assistant, who will collect and condense information for presentation. Legislative assistants frequently determine whether issues are presented favorably or unfavorably, and can have substantial influence over policy decisions. Be respectful and courteous; you may gain an ally and knowledgeable resource.[13]

Face to Face

Meeting a legislator can be intimidating, but remember that *you* are the *health care expert*. Be polite, but confident. Dress professionally, arrive early, and wait patiently. Occasionally, you may end up meeting with a legislative assistant, instead; treat him with the same courtesy you would give the legislator. When you meet the legislator, follow the same format suggested for written communication. Introduce yourself and shake hands. State where you are from, whether you are a constituent, and if you are representing a group. Explain what you want from the legislator, tell your story, give pertinent facts, repeat your request, and entertain questions. Take a few notes; come prepared, but be flexible and attempt to have a normal and open conversation. Maintain a pleasant, professional tone and do not become derogatory or defensive. Try to frame your position in positive terms and portray yourself as *for* an issue rather than *against* an opposing view.[13] Be respectful of your legislator's time, thank her at the close of the conversation, and indicate you will follow up on your request. Leave your contact information and indicate your availability for further conversation regarding your issue; offer to testify before a committee.

Testifying Before Committee

The experience of giving testimony before a legislative committee tends to be more structured than individual meetings and is guided by the committee chairman, but the same basic principles of etiquette and self-presentation apply. Professional business attire is appropriate. When you arrive, let the chairman know you are there. When asked to testify, start by introducing yourself, explaining your credentials, and stating whether you are for or against the specific bill in question; then make your case as you normally would. Visual aids, PowerPoints, and handouts are unnecessary, but you may wish to bring notes for yourself. It may be worthwhile to prepare both short and long versions of your statement in order to adapt to changeable time allotments. Be prepared for distraction; committee members may speak to each other, pass notes, or read other documents. Regardless, if they ask a question, assume they are paying attention and answer it. Finally, be prepared to testify before multiple committees.

WHEN TO MAKE CONTACT

Search out unique opportunities for meeting with legislators. Attend ACEP's annual *Leadership and Advocacy Conference* in Washington D.C. every May, the ACEP state chapter legislative conferences, or coordinate a legislative day with state chapters of specialty societies. Some congressmen return home to their districts during weekends, which may provide time to schedule a meeting.[13] As your legislation progresses, your activities and contacts may shift as well. When proposing a bill, reach out to legislators who might sponsor and champion your cause.[5] When a bill is in committee, offer testimony on the record.[16] Contact your legislators again when legislation is coming to a vote. This process can be prolonged and requires persistence; but, maintaining contact can create long-term liaisons for continued cooperation on future projects.

FUTURE AVENUES FOR ADVOCACY: SOCIAL MEDIA

The exponential growth of social media outlets such as Facebook, YouTube, Flickr, and Twitter has redefined the political landscape and opened new avenues for political participation and advocacy. For example, the Obama campaign successfully used social media in the 2008 election to produce record turnouts among minority youth voters.[19] Recognizing its growing importance, political parties are using dedicated social media teams to create Facebook pages for national conventions, stream caucus meetings, and blog full-time.[20]

Many advocacy websites offer Facebook or Twitter links with daily updates on public health topics. Engaging in participatory politics through web-based social media transcends simply moving institutional political activity to an online format. You can organize a political demonstration via Facebook, write your own blog about political candidates or campaigns, or post a political video on YouTube. The skills and networks citizens develop by using social media to engage in socializing and sharing interests are being translated to the political realm, allowing individuals to cheaply and easily mobilize groups and reach ever-larger audiences through social networks.[21]

ADVOCACY AS SCHOLARSHIP

Share your efforts with the academic community. Scholarly publications on advocacy remain relatively scarce. Advocacy often does not fit in the traditional scholarship model and typically has not been promoted through the academic rewards of faculty promotion or tenure. Opponents of increased calls for advocacy in the medical profession even argue that advocacy may *subvert* academic scholarship, "as advocacy seeks change rather than knowledge."[22]

Models for scholarly advocacy *do* exist, however. Influential American educator, Ernest Boyer, PhD, proposed an alternative model in which advocacy may be considered the "scholarship of *application*," alongside the more traditional scholarship of *discovery*.[23] Publish your experience and work in advocacy; your colleagues will learn through your successes and failures. As advocacy becomes increasingly integral to the medical profession, physicians need to be recognized for their expertise, and their advocacy efforts need to be acknowledged for what they are – true scholarly pursuits.

CONCLUSION

As long as emergency departments remain the canary in our current health care coal mine, emergency physicians will be ideally situated to advocate for the health of both individual patients and communities. Advocacy can take many forms. Find your passion and use the information and strategies in this handbook to speak up for your specialty, whether on a local or national scale. Be patient, be persistent, and continue to serve as your patients' voice. ✶

HOW A BILL BECOMES A LAW

Jamie "Akiva" Kahn, MD, MBA

While the words of Schoolhouse Rock's catchy tune, "I'm Just a Bill," may have faded from our childhood memories, the image of the weary bill "sitting here on Capitol Hill" has endured.[1] The song provided, for many of us, a glimpse into how an idea becomes a bill – and, potentially, a law. While this process is relatively straight-forward, it is important to understand the chain of events that leads to legislation; as health care providers who advocate for bills in motion, it is critical to know and speak the language of the legislative process.

RESEARCH AND WRITING OF A BILL

Any individual or group of individuals is permitted to write a bill. The ability of the general populace to take part in the lawmaking process is just a portion of what forms our "democratic republic." First, appropriate research must be conducted into what current laws exist and how they may affect a bill, or if changes to current legislation are needed. After that, the bill must be written and introduced to Congress. For introduction, the assistance of a member of the Senate or House of Representatives (or assembly, in some states) is needed.

Find a Legislator to Sponsor Your Idea

The decision about which legislator should introduce and represent a particular bill is vitally important; that person must be well-respected and have a clear understanding of and an interest in the proposed legislation. It is also helpful to select a legislator who serves on the committee to which a bill may be assigned, as he or she will be able to shepherd it through the process.

Introduction of the Bill

The legislator who agrees to sponsor the bill then introduces it to either the House or Senate (with the exception of Nebraska, which is a one-house legislative system), where the bill is received by the clerk and assigned a number. After the introduction of a bill, the Speaker of the House or Senate President will send it to a committee with the appropriate jurisdiction; the bill may then be sent to a subcommittee, if deemed necessary.

Committee Consideration

Within the committees and subcommittees, hearings may be held, wherein witnesses testify about the benefits and consequences of enacting the bill. Bills often "die in committee" and never receive a formal hearing or vote. The process by which legislation is officially reviewed, and possibly amended, occurs during the "mark-up." When a mark-up is completed (with or without changes), the committee or subcommittee votes on a final draft of the bill. The committee may then decide to sit on the bill and eliminate it from further consideration (otherwise known as *tabling*), defeat the measure, or recommend it be "reported out" of committee. If a subcommittee approves the measure, the bill is presented to the *full* committee, where it will go through the same steps and consideration process as it did in the subcommittee.

Full Chamber Consideration

When the bill is approved by the full committee(s), it must be placed on the House or Senate calendar for debate by the full chamber. At that time, it can be debated and amended (depending on the rules accompanying the legislation) by the entire chamber. At the state level, this process can be highly variable; knowledge of parliamentary procedures is crucial for ensuring that the bill is not defeated on technical grounds. The full chamber can table the bill, refer it back to committee (if it is not satisfied with the bill as written), or it can choose to either defeat or approve the measure.

Second House Consideration

After a bill passes one House of Congress, it must then be sent to the other house for consideration. At times, two similar bills may be submitted simultaneously to both houses for review and consideration. Most notably, the recent health reform bill was submitted in two similar forms – one to the U.S. Senate and one to the U.S. House of Representatives.

There are three ways that a bill can be approved and move on to the executive branch:

1. The second chamber approves the bill without making any amendments;
2. Amendments made by the second house are sent back and approved by the first chamber without further modification; or
3. The two chambers disagree on amendments added and a conference committee is formed (usually with members of both houses) to write the conference report. The bill is then sent back to both chambers for a final vote. If both chambers approve the conference report, it will be sent to the governor or the president.

BECOMING A LAW

Pursuant to *Article 1, Section 7* of the U.S. Constitution, "Every Bill, which shall have passed the House of Representatives and the Senate, shall, before it become a Law, be presented to the President of the United States; . . ." The president has four options after the identical bill passes both houses of the legislature:

1. **Sign the bill into law (enactment).** The process of signing the bill often is a time for political "theater," with signing ceremonies and celebratory presidential pens passed out to key advocates.
2. **Veto the bill.** If the bill is vetoed, it is returned – along with a veto message – to the legislative branch. The bill can still be passed into law (veto override) if it receives a two-thirds vote in both the House and the Senate. Veto override is one example of *checks-and-balances*, which enables one branch of government to limit the powers of the other branches.

3. **Take no action while Congress is in session.** After a specified number of days (10 in federal legislation), the bill will become law without signature.
4. **Pocket veto.** Take no action and allow the Congress to adjourn (only if fewer than 10 days remain between the bill's passage in Congress and adjournment). This is known as a *pocket veto*; the bill cannot return to Congress and it expires, effectively killing it.[23]

REGULATORY IMPLEMENTATION

Many think of the president's signature as the last step in the development of a bill. Congress often will give broad targets and funding for parts of the legislation, but will leave the details to the administrative process. While each administrative body is different, the fundamental path of implementation is similar. The governing administrative agency will develop rules for implementation; these rules will then be published for comment and review by the public for a defined time period. After all comments have been reviewed, the administrative body will publish its final rules. The need for regulatory advocacy is present at all stages of the development, comment, and implementation of the legislation.

ATYPICAL ROUTE OF BILL DEVELOPMENT

Health care reform demonstrated that the simple process described above may, in fact, be far more complex. In the summer of 2009, three Democratic and three Republican Senate Finance Committee members, Senators Max Baucus (D-Montana), Chuck Grassley (R-Iowa), Kent Conrad (D-North Dakota), Olympia Snowe (R-Maine), Jeff Bingaman (D-New Mexico), and Mike Enzi (R-Wyoming), met extensively to discuss what became the foundation of the Senate's health care reform bill, but the Senate did not immediately introduce a bill following these negotiations. On November 7, 2009, the House of Representatives passed the first health care reform bill, entitled the "Affordable Health Care for America Act," with a 220 to 215 vote.[5] This bill was forwarded to the Senate for consideration, but the Senate declined to debate it; the senators instead developed a bill of their own based on their earlier bipartisan discussions. As the Republican minority vowed to filibuster any bill they did not support, 60 Senate votes were required for a cloture vote to end debate and pass the bill.

After extensive negotiations to build the 60 vote majority, the Affordable Care Act (ACA) of 2010 was passed on December 24, 2009.[6] House Democrats noted many differences between the ACA and their November 2009 legislation and were unwilling to pass the ACA without several changes. In order to continue the progress of the legislation, House Democrats ultimately did pass the Senate's health care reform bill (the ACA) along with Health Care and Education Reconciliation Act of 2010 (the "reconciliation bill") in March 2010. The Senate approved the amendments by reconciliation, and the ACA was signed into law by President Obama by the end of March 2010.[7]

JUDICIAL CHECKS AND BALANCES

The health care reform bill also demonstrated the importance of the third branch of government, the judiciary. Since being signed into law, the constitutionality of certain portions the bill have been questioned by groups, which oppose its various provisions. On the day the law was enacted, 26 states, several individuals, and others sued to have the law struck down. Most of the suits challenge the legal standing of the individual mandate. Opponents argued that it violates the commerce clause by requiring citizens to purchase health insurance or pay a "shared responsibility payment" to the government, thus infringing upon a person's freedom to choose how to spend his or her own health care dollars. Other suits are based around different components of the ACA, including Medicaid expansion, the Independent Physician Advisory Board, the penalty for not buying insurance, the possibility of federal funding for abortion, and medical privacy.

On June 28, 2012, the United States Supreme Court upheld the constitutionality of the ACA in the *National Federation of Independent Business v. Sebelius* case; it was argued that the individual mandate was a tax, therefore a constitutional application of Congress's taxation power.[8] Since being ruled constitutional, the House of Representatives has made numerous attempts to repeal the bill.[9]

CONCLUSION

Understanding the legislative process – and where and how to be involved – is critical to being an effective advocate. While health care reform recently has shown us that the process is not nearly as simple as the song we learned as children, the need for advocacy has never been more important. ✶

With thanks to Donald Ross Patrick Jr., MD, for his authorship of a previous version of this chapter.

Federal Government Resources
- The White House: http://www.whitehouse.gov
- United States House of Representatives: http://www.house.gov
- United States Senate: http://senate.gov
- Library of Congress (Thomas): http://thomas.loc.gov
- United States Supreme Court: http://www.supremecourt.gov

State and Local Government Resources
- National Conference of State Legislatures: http://www.ncsl.org
- U.S. Department of States: http://www.America.gov

Health Care Reform Resources
- http://www.healthcare.gov
- http://www.whitehouse.gov/healthreform

Chapter 21

PEOPLE AND ORGANIZATIONS IN ADVOCACY

Ashley Ryles, MD and Nathaniel R. Schlicher, MD, JD, FACEP

Advocacy, while effective on an individual basis, often is better achieved when people join forces for a common purpose. There are many organizations that work toward improving care for emergency department patients and providers. Regardless of which group you choose, it is important to be a part of a *club*. Work across organizations is needed to advance programs and defend against potentially damaging policies; knowing with whom to connect will help advance your goals and benefit your patients.

Advocacy opportunities within the organization include:

EMRA

The *Emergency Medicine Residents' Association* (EMRA) was founded in 1974 and today has more than 11,000 members. It ranks as the second-largest specialty association in emergency medicine, behind the American College of Emergency Physicians (ACEP), and is the oldest and largest independent resident organization in the world. With its own operating budget and leadership, the issues of residents remain the focus of its every action. The organization works collaboratively with ACEP on common goals and projects, under a shared services agreement, but retains its independent spirit in all aspects.

Legislative Advisor

EMRA's legislative advisor position was created to serve on the organization's board of directors and help with legal, political, and administrative issues. With the ever-changing nature of health care delivery, those serving in this role advise members on current advocacy issues and educate them on laws that impact the practice of medicine. The position gradually has changed over the past five years. Initially an appointed position to the EMRA Board of Directors, it became a fully elected position at-large in 2010. Like most board positions, any resident member may apply and campaign for it.

Health Policy Committee

Recognizing that no *one* individual could perform the task of marshaling all legislative issues, EMRA created its Health Policy Committee in 2008. The committee was founded to support the board on health policy issues affecting its members. This position is ideal for residents interested in health policy, politics, or legislation. EMRA committee members were instrumental in the development of the first edition of the *Advocacy Handbook* and the Advocacy Lecture Series.

LAC

The *Leadership and Advocacy Conference* (LAC) was created by ACEP to help train and develop leaders in the practice of emergency medicine. Politicians make legislative decisions (such as EMTALA) that have a long-lasting impact on the practice of medicine. Each physician must be an active voice in the political process as fundamental changes in the nature of health care delivery are discussed. This conference is an opportunity for physicians to get training in political advocacy to help further the goals of delivering high-quality emergency medical services. One day of the conference, which is hosted in Washington D.C., is dedicated to making visits to legislators' offices on Capitol Hill to educate and influence elected leaders on important issues in emergency medicine.

EMRA hosts a portion of LAC that is specifically tailored to the interests of residents and first-time conference attendees. With a track that involves lectures, advocacy training, and receptions with leaders in the specialty, the conference has continued to provide a unique educational opportunity for resident physicians. EMRA annually issues its *Chair's Challenge,* a call for residency program chairs to sponsor their residents' LAC attendance. With a nominal registration fee for EMRA members of $25, each resident can attend for little more than the costs of transportation and housing.

ACEP

With more than 31,000 members, the *American College of Emergency Physicians* (ACEP) is the largest emergency medicine specialty organization in the United States. The college's formation coincided with the establishment of the specialty to represent the interests of emergency physicians and help develop the field. Today, the organization is active across the legislative, regulatory, and administrative spectrum to help advance the interests of its members and patients.

Emergency Medicine Practice Management and Health Policy Section

The *Emergency Medicine Practice Management and Health Policy Section* is one of 32 sections of membership within ACEP. It provides members a forum for sharing ideas and experiences in order to effectively manage critical and emerging public policy issues.

ACEP Committees

ACEP's *Federal Governmental Affairs Committee* and the *State Legislative and Regulatory Committee* are groups within the organization that work on issues regarding advocacy. Any member of ACEP (including EMRA members) may apply to serve on a committee. The president-elect chooses committee members to serve during his or her presidential year. While some committees are very competitive, there is always space for passionate advocates to be involved within the organization.

THE 911 NETWORK

Emergency medicine physicians treat patients in their greatest times of need; as such, they bear witness to the health care system's greatest successes and most tragic failings. Despite the passage of the ACA, immense work still is needed on the regulatory issues and ongoing potential legislative reforms. Knowledge of the local and national health care agenda is critical to powerful advocacy. The ACEP 911 Network is one of the easiest ways to become a better-informed physician and more effective advocate, and brings together over 1,400 ACEP and EMRA members. ACEP established the network in 1998 to encourage members to cultivate long-term relationships with federal legislators, convey legislative and regulatory priorities and affect the final outcome of federal legislation important to emergency medicine.

The ACEP 911 Network offers several avenues for advocacy participation:

- **Weekly Updates.** Sent by e-mail to inform participants of the latest legislative, political, and regulatory issues and activities.
- **Action Alerts.** Sent by email, requesting members to contact their U.S. representatives or senators about a specific issue or vote.
- **Delivery of NEMPAC Contributions.** Some NEMPAC contributions are delivered directly by 911 Network members who reside in the legislators' districts.
- **ED Visits.** Members are encouraged to invite legislators to tour their emergency departments. This provides legislators and their staff the opportunity to witness first-hand the operations of an ED and to meet their constituents.
- **Team Captains.** The ACEP 911 Network is organized by a group of team captains who receive focused training and communications, increased resources, and special recognition for their efforts.
- **Advocacy Training.** Members of the 911 Network are encouraged to continually develop their advocacy skills. To help improve lobbying efforts, political education training is offered each year during ACEP's Leadership and Advocacy Conference and *Scientific Assembly* (SA). These programs are designed to help physician members learn more about the federal legislative process and effective grassroots lobbying techniques.

EDPMA

The *Emergency Department Practice Management Association* (EDPMA) was founded in 1997 to represent the interests and concerns of emergency medicine physicians with members of Congress and the Centers for Medicare and Medicaid (CMS), while empowering members with information on both legislative and regulatory issues facing the specialty. Its members include emergency medicine physician groups and national organizations.

NEMPAC

The *National Emergency Medicine Political Action Committee* (NEMPAC) is a critical advocacy powerhouse, which augments the voice of emergency physicians and their patients in the federal election process. National political action committees (or PACs) combine donations from individuals to make meaningful contributions to federal candidates running for a seats in the U.S. House of Representatives or Senate.

As physicians, our success as advocates hinges upon our ability to work with federal lawmakers who share a common vision to improve emergency services. Because health care is at the top of the priority list for many candidates, contributions to NEMPAC will help facilitate the emergency physician's place at the table. In recent years, NEMPAC contributions to political campaigns have focused on candidates who support emergency medicine reform issues like the *Access to Emergency Medical Services Act*.

In addition, NEMPAC continues to push for legislation to increase the number of emergency medicine residency positions funded by the federal government, and supports proposals that would defer student loan payments until after residency and fellowship training is complete. Simply put, the mission of NEMPAC is to use campaign contributions and political advocacy to support candidates that foster the legislative priorities of emergency medicine patients and physicians. Based on the 2012 election cycle, NEMPAC is the fourth largest physician specialty political action committee. In the 2012 elections, NEMPAC donated more than $2 million to a total of 238 candidates for the House and Senate.

EMAF

The *Emergency Medicine Action Fund* was established in 2011 to complement the work of NEMPAC. While PAC funds contribute directly to candidates and affect the legislative process, the goal of EMAF is to influence regulatory processes. This is done through tax-deductible activities, such as convening high-level meetings with regulatory agencies, commissioning studies to quantify the value of emergency medicine, and examining and evaluating new practice models (including bundled payments and ACOs). EMAF contributors include key emergency medicine organizations such as EMRA, ACEP, CORD, SAEM, AAEM and ACOEP, as well as many other physician groups and coalitions. In its inaugural year, EMAF supported research and provided direct funding to Washington state for legal challenges related to the flawed policy regarding limitations on perceived non-emergent visits. This was an early and significant victory for the new organization.

STATE-LEVEL ADVOCACY

State medical associations, as well as state chapters of ACEP, offer unique opportunities to get involved in advocacy on a more localized level. State medical associations are coalitions of physicians that work across specialty lines to help improve working conditions for physicians within an individual state. Local state medical board websites can provide information on getting involved and developing an understanding of the needs of physicians, patients, and communities. Many state medical societies – and some state chapters of ACEP – convene an annual *advocacy day*, which is similar to LAC, but hosted at the state capitol. Additionally, state ACEP chapter leaders often can help arrange guest lectures on important health policy issues in an individual area.

ADVOCACY PROGRAMS

There are multiple opportunities available for getting more involved in the advocacy process – from short stays to year-long programs.

ACEP/EMRA Mini-Fellowship. This is a month-long opportunity to experience advocacy at the national level. The program is supported by EMRA and ACEP with the goal of training future leaders and introducing them to the advocacy process. Mini-fellows spend a month at ACEP's public affairs office in Washington D.C., usually as an elective during their residencies. During this time, ample opportunities are provided to meet with legislators, attend committee hearings and educational sessions, and assist with the critical advocacy work of the D.C. office.

Advocacy Fellowships. There are multiple non-ACGME approved advocacy fellowships, which generally are one year in duration. Programs involve advocacy work on local and national levels, in additional to clinical shifts. Use the EMRA "match" page (www.emra/match) to locate ongoing advocacy programs explore their curricula. Currently available fellowships include:

- ACEP California Chapter – *Health Policy & Advocacy Fellowship*
- George Washington University – *Health Policy Fellowship*
- Oregon Health & Science University – *Research Fellowship*
- University of Illinois at Chicago – *International Fellowship*
- UT Southwestern Medical Center – *Practice Management and Health Policy Fellowship*
- UCLA – *Robert Wood Johnson Foundation Clinical Scholars Program*

Robert Wood Johnson Foundation Health Policy Fellowship. Initiated in 1973, the Robert Wood Johnson Foundation Health Policy Fellows program is a comprehensive 12-month fellowship experience at the nexus of health science, policy, and politics in Washington, D.C. Fellows participate in the policy process at the federal level and use that leadership experience to improve health, health care and health policy. During these assignments, fellows contribute to the policy process with members of Congress and will help develop legislative proposals, arrange hearings, meet with constituents, brief legislators for committee sessions and floor debates, and staff House-Senate conferences.

WEB ADVOCACY RESOURCES

A number of online advocacy resources are available, which provide the tools necessary to reach out to representatives and develop effective advocacy skills.

www.EMRA.org

The website offers a fully accessible repository of advocacy articles and topics. The original Advocacy Lecture Series also is available for download and modification.

www.ACEP.org

The ACEP website represents one of the premier emergency medicine professional societies. The "Advocacy" tab lays out a number of important concepts for young physician advocates, including detailed explanations of the ACEP 911 Network, NEMPAC, and the Leadership and Advocacy Conference.

www.AMA.org

The American Medical Association offers a number of programs designed to help physicians develop advocacy skills. These include conferences focused on advising and organizing political campaigns, for those interested in pursuing political office.

CONCLUSION

Regardless of the organization in which you choose to be involved, it is crucial to the ongoing success and growth of emergency medicine for every resident to be informed and involved in the legal, regulatory, political, and administrative issues that will affect them and the care of their patients. We hope that you choose to join EMRA in advancing the cause of emergency medicine and excellent patient care. ✶

Chapter 22

BUILDING AN ADVOCACY COALITION

Brooke L. Donaldson, MD

Ask any emergency medicine physician what makes our environment unique and you will get a variety of answers. From the need to make split-second life and death decisions, to the atmosphere of the ED, to our challenging patient population, ours is a distinguished specialty. Emergency medicine often is described as a "family," and it is difficult for those outside the field to fully understand what we do and why. Our specialty is a coalition of like-minded individuals working towards patient advocacy; however, it is often difficult for any single group of individuals to accomplish its goals alone within the complex political landscape in which we operate. The ability to build coalitions and support is necessary to achieve change.

DEFINITION

A *coalition* is "a combination or alliance; a union into one body or mass."[2] Coalitions can be formal, such as the American Medical Association; or informal, such as a group of emergency physicians working at a particular hospital. A coalition is a format for organizations to "effectively harness and focus" a collection of resources.[2] It is the simple choice of uniting to achieve a common goal. Emergency medicine physicians work together to provide the best possible care for patients every day. They also work with the hospital administration to set policies that make this goal a reality. This is the simplest form of a coalition.

The long-term success of the coalition is not based on which path it takes; but, rather, on the group's ability to maintain and renew the vitality, passion, and commitment that was present on day one.

The details of the coalition follow the goals and structure of its members. It can be large or small, formal or informal, government-based or independent. A *government-based* coalition, an organization with a formal governance structure, is "a governing body formed by multiple parties who must compromise on principles" in order to achieve a desired outcome.[3] Agencies, such as the American Medical Association (AMA) and American Heart Association (AHA), are examples of such coalitions. These agencies team with independent groups and individual health care providers to address government policy and affect changes that will benefit both providers and patients.

EXAMPLES OF COALITIONS

The AMA is one of the largest coalitions available to physicians. Its mission is to "promote the art and science of medicine and the betterment of public health."[5] The AMA is comprised of physicians from around the country who support the organization's cause, core values, and mission. The degree of involvement in the coalition varies among members; some are financial supporters, while others serve on committees, and still others represent the coalition as advocates in Washington, D.C. The AMA is a prime example of a national coalition that unites the broader health care society in order to improve the professional lives of physicians and patients by influencing public policy.

While the AMA has an extensive scope, some coalitions are formed for a specific cause and focuse solely on that purpose. *Protect Patients Now* (PPN) is one such coalition. It is an advocacy association whose principal intent is to "reform our nation's broken medical liability system."[6] PPN is a branch of the *Health Coalition on Liability and Access* (HCLA) and represents health care consumers, health care providers, hospitals, insurers, and businesses. Its members believe the current liability system does not adequately protect patients and does not keep them at the forefront. The organization's mission is to reform the current system by improving "access and innovation" and discouraging "defensive medicine."[6] This coalition has a strictly defined platform, goals, and objectives.

BUILDING YOUR ADVOCACY COALITION

The most important step in building your own advocacy coalition is defining its intent. Once you have defined your purpose, you must consider the suitability of a coalition for the particular cause. Is a formal coalition obligatory to sustain a noticeable change? Are there other operational organizations that already are serving the same cause? Would these organizations' resources be better utilized in an allied group? Are there others who share the same views and opinions? Is the issue a priority to the target audience?

Once the final decision to configure a coalition has been made, the process of forming it begins. This is a multistep process for which there are many approaches.

After declaring the *intent* of your coalition, you must analyze its potential risks, demands, and the currently available resources. This analysis will serve as your organization's foundation. It will focus and direct the group toward establishing a cohesive action plan; it is your first step.

Next, from the information obtained in your initial cause determination and analysis, you will be ready to identify and establish specific principles, objectives, and goals for the coalition. These initially should be ascertained by the primary leadership of the coalition; however, they should be stated in such a way that they are flexible to the overall needs and desires of the membership as a whole. Once the goals, objectives, and principles are created, they should be presented to the membership at large for discussion and acceptance. It is critical for these to be uncontroversial and widely accepted by all members; this will provide dividends by reducing future disagreements.[1,4]

Success in these early steps will improve the credibility, motivation, funding, and volunteerism within the coalition. The longevity of the group also needs to be determined in the early planning stages. Will the coalition end after completion of its objectives, after the legislative term, or at the end of a defined period of time? Or is the goal – and therefore the coalition – an ongoing endeavor? This also may change over the course of the coalition's actions, as the problems and solutions are presented and the need for ongoing advocacy is further identified.

Finally, the last step of the coalition's foundation is deciding its name. It is imperative to name the coalition based on the *issue* for which it represents rather than on the priorities of a particular organization. This will peak the interest of the largest number of members and financial supporters.[1,4]

LEADERSHIP, MEMBERSHIP, AND FINANCES WITHIN THE COALITION

The coalition's leadership and membership are pivotal to its survival and success. The leadership team can be structured in a variety of ways: a *chairperson*, a *steering committee*, or an *overseeing organization*. When deciding who should assume these roles, it is important to consider the tasks that will become their primary responsibilities. These include, but are not limited to: initial formation of the coalition, management, communication amongst members and supporters, fiscal and fiduciary responsibilities, obtaining resources, and facilitating consensus and cohesiveness. The leadership team ultimately needs to have the power, vision, knowledge, and communication skills to establish and renew the coalition and its enthusiasts.[1,4]

The principles, objectives, and goals are the *foundation* of the coalition, while the leadership team is the *mortar* that holds the coalition together. Consequently, the members serve as the *infrastructure* that keeps the coalition standing. Membership should embody a diverse group of people with multidimensional interests, talents, skills, temperaments, and involvement. By creating a comprehensive membership, the coalition can be publicized as a "broad, social movement" with a defined cause, rather than being labeled as a "narrow sectarian cause."[1] Coalition members offer more than just support; they also provide professional expertise, financial backing, political and media-related access, and geographic representation. With a diverse membership, it is important to remain true to the foundation on which the coalition was built, unless the entire group compromises on a splinter issue.[1,4]

The coalition's core message is used not only to gain membership, but also for advertisement purposes and to secure financial sponsorship. Finances are a difficult, but crucial, part of any coalition's survival. With a clear message and a stable foundation, financial resources can be sought. Membership fees are a primary source of funding and can be used for startup capital or for ongoing operations. Grants and corporate contributions can be sought for selected causes, but can be time-intensive and difficult to obtain. The goals of your individual coalition will determine your financial needs.[1,4]

Now that you have established your coalition, it is important to continue to reassess its progress and vitality. Trials and tribulations will be faced; you can anticipate unproductive meetings, bureaucracy vexation, alterations of goals, members with poorly defined roles, and displeasure with current scenarios along the way. It should be a priority of the leadership team to foresee and quickly diffuse as many of these problems as possible. The long-term success of the coalition is not based on which path it takes; but, rather, on the group's ability to maintain and renew the vitality, passion, and commitment that was present on day one.

THE WHO, WHAT, AND WHEN OF AN ESTABLISHED COALITION

In Washington State, the Health Care Authority (which governs Medicaid) released a plan to reduce "unnecessary" emergency department visits by retrospective analysis of patients' final discharge diagnoses. The Washington Chapter of the American College of Emergency Physicians, Washington State Medical Association, and Washington State Hospital Association identified the issue as a problem with "perceived overuse of hospital EDs by Medicaid patients."[7] They formed a coalition to "address the real 'root of the problem.'"[7] This became their foundation and the coalition's message.

Although these groups could have addressed the problem individually, their united front allowed them to better utilize their resources and propose a solution that benefited all involved. This is a *true* coalition. An issue was identified (the foundation of the coalition); several organizations united as one (the leadership and membership); and they worked together to provide a positive outcome (the goal).

Much like many other coalitions, the need for this one has continued beyond the original framework. The coalition is now expanding in Washington State to include other organizations and groups, such as primary care providers, to address additional challenges and tangential issues. These changes can induce growing pains, but often strengthen the organization and increase their chances of future success.

CONCLUSION

A coalition is a powerful instrument that synergizes a diverse group of individuals, allowing them to collectively focus their efforts to create effective, positive change. A successful infrastructure can be built by appropriately identifying the principles, goals, and objectives that will comprise the coalition's message; creating an efficient leadership team; and building the commitment of the group's members. By working *together* toward a common goal, individuals, organizations, and groups can have greater influence on the subject than they could ever have achieved single-handedly. ✶

Chapter 23

STATE AND LOCAL ADVOCACY

Robert Cooper, MD, MPH and Eric Cortez, MD

THE IMPORTANCE OF STATE AND LOCAL ADVOCACY

While much of our country's recent health care reform debate has occurred at the national level, states are equally influential in enacting change. The executive and legislative branches of state governments play vital roles in professional licensure, continuing medical education requirements, malpractice and tort reform, physician reimbursement, and loan forgiveness.[1] Additionally, many federal programs are enacted at the state level, with significant local discretion regarding their implementation; Medicaid is an example of a large *hybrid* state and federal program.

THE STATE LEGISLATIVE PROCESS

State governments are structured much like the federal government and consist of *executive, legislative,* and *judicial* branches. The governor and lieutenant governor head the executive branch; other officials include the attorney general, secretary of state, auditors, and commissioners. The state legislature consists of senators and representatives who may be either full-time or part-time. Every state has a dual-chamber legislature, except for Nebraska, which has one chamber. In all states, the smaller chamber is referred to as the Senate and, in most states, the larger chamber is referred to as the House of Representatives.[2]

State senators serve four-year terms and are led by the senate president. House and Assembly members serve two-year terms and are led by the speaker of the house. Each chamber has committees to which legislators are assigned, based on party affiliation, personal interest, and district representation.[2]

Bills typically are introduced by legislators through specific committees. The bill proposals are then debated in each chamber and passed. Differences between the two chambers must be reconciled and then presented to the governor;[3] the governor can either sign the bill into law or veto it. Depending on the majority vote, the legislature can pass a bill despite veto by the governor; and, even after a bill has passed, the executive branch must develop policies and procedures for its implementation.[3]

ADVOCACY STRATEGIES AT THE STATE LEVEL

Successful advocacy begins with recognizing our responsibility to advocate for our patients and society. The American College of Emergency Physicians declares advocacy an *ethical duty*, extending from the responsibilities society grants us as physicians.[4] So important is this role, emergency medicine leaders are being called to consider advocacy a scholarly endeavor and cause for promotion and tenure in academic settings, as well.[3]

In the book *Good to Great*, author Jim Collins describes three essential elements to success in any endeavor: *passion, skill*, and a *clear, well-defined goal*.[5] These same elements apply to advocacy at the state level.

Possessing enough *passion* about an issue to advocate for change seems simple; however, when faced with the demands of a stressful job, family, and continuing medical education, this passion often is neglected. Developing and nurturing a passion for emergency medicine outside of day-to-day shift work, through activities such as advocacy, can greatly increase an emergency physician's career satisfaction.

Skilled advocates demonstrate a strong understanding of the issues and know how to communicate with the right people.[6] Emergency physicians witness the trials and tribulations that patients face every day without health insurance or access to primary care. We understand the shortcomings of EMTALA. In essence, we are uniquely positioned to provide testimony to state legislators. State advocacy requires much more than anecdotal experiences, however; being knowledgeable also means understanding the benefits and consequences of your cause. Advocates must present evidence, research studies, and statistics to reinforce their arguments.[6]

Skilled advocates also are effective communicators.[6] While the *means* vary and depend on numerous circumstances, direct and understandable communication is always most effective when advocating for a cause.[6] Although the presentation of extensive evidence and supporting research is important, many feel the most effective communication method is *storytelling*. Policymakers tend to remember compelling stories and anecdotes better than they do statistics, and are more inclined to respond in a positive manner.[7] The patient who has been directly affected by a particular piece of legislation will have greater influence on lawmakers than a stack of numbers.

Successful advocates are *goal-oriented*. Specific, well-defined outcomes are better than generalizations.[5] A specific task, whether it be a piece of legislation, a letter to a regulatory agency or other intervention, is critical. This kind of targeted advocacy provides a much better chance of success than the expression of general concern without a specific action plan. A *clear task* is required to ensure that your passion and skills are working together toward a specific goal.[6]

EXAMPLES OF EFFECTIVE STATE ADVOCACY

There are many recent examples of successful state advocacy led by emergency physicians. In 2003, West Virginia and Florida enacted bills addressing EMTALA-related tort reform; two years later, Georgia and South Carolina passed similar bills.[8] Texas' Proposition 12, which capped non-economic damages, led to a 70% reduction in the number of lawsuits filed against hospitals in the state, and an 8% decrease in malpractice liability premiums;[9] the legislation also has reduced malpractice claims by nearly 50%.[10]

In recent years, the Ohio ACEP chapter has championed EMTALA-related tort reform in its state. The organization introduced Senate Bill 86, *Access to Emergency Care and Disaster Care,* to advance medical liability reform.

Obtaining Contacts and Sponsors

Most lawmakers are experts in whatever fields they worked prior to entering the legislature; they often have backgrounds in law or business, and – very rarely – medicine. Their unfamiliarity with emergency medicine makes legislators susceptible to common misconceptions about the specialty, including high health care costs, drug-seeking behavior, and long wait times. Led by Dr. Gary Katz, the Ohio ACEP team began by showing the lawmakers the realities of emergency medicine using statistical data from reputable sources, such as the Centers for Disease Control.

These crucial informational meetings were only were made possible by the years of relationship-building and political advocacy prior to the introduction of SB 86.[11] Relationship-building centers on "pounding the pavement"; it is much easier to call a legislator if you're already on a first-name basis. Developing of this personal relationship may require attending fundraisers, meeting your legislators at the state house, and inviting them to visit your emergency department. If you can avoid being the person who is always asking for something; the lawmaker will be more likely to listen when you really *do* need something.

Legislators are most amenable to being approached by one of their constituents. Even when a leader of an organization is going to a meeting, it is important to bring a physician-constituent prepared on the key talking points to each meeting with local lawmakers. Regular calls for advocacy and membership updates will help keep the issue alive in the local district. The Ohio ACEP newsletter always began with a key action item, such as letter writing or a call for donations in or der to help members focus on what steps to take to help move the bill forward.

Lobbying and Bill Preparation

It is difficult to get a bill introduced – let alone *passed* – without employing a lobbying firm. Lobbyists are familiar with individual lawmakers and their agendas. Not only do they know whom to approach, they also have long relationships with many lawmakers, making it easier to secure meetings and support. With the help of a lobbyist, the Ohio ACEP chapter identified key legislators, focusing on those who expressed an understanding of their concerns about medical liability and patient's access to care, regardless of their position on the political spectrum.[11]

After identifying lawmakers who might support EMTALA-related tort reform, Ohio ACEP sat down to actually write the bill. While the goals of the bill already were established, the Ohio organization used the aforementioned bills from Florida and Texas to establish the actual language for its own. Lawmakers often refer to nationally known bills such as these as precedents, so it is important to use the pre-existing language to provide a similar framework.

One area where Ohio ACEP encountered trouble in writing SB 86 was in the Legislative Services Committee (LSC). The LSC is a non-partisan committee that assures compliance of all proposed legislation with Ohio Revised Code. The LSC initially provided an edited version of SB 86 that would have conflicted with EMTALA; this led Ohio ACEP to recognize the importance of educating the LSC members about emergency medicine by providing ED site visits.[11]

Gaining Support and Anticipating Opposition

To gain support from other subspecialties, Ohio ACEP made clear that SB 86 was about improving access to emergency care, not just about tort reform. The organization emphasized that many non-academic medical centers do not have access to on-call specialists. They cited statistics regarding the risk and costs of transport to tertiary care centers, and emphasized that liability costs reduce the likelihood of specialists taking emergency calls. While most in-hospital specialists and their professional organizations quickly supported the bill, the primary care community was slower to demonstrate support. The Ohio ACEP physicians presented their data at regional primary care and individual practice meetings; eventually, the primary care community offered its support of the bill, as well.[11]

Oho ACEP identified early on that trial attorneys would be the primary opposition. The attorneys argued that SB 86 would lead to declining quality of care and denial of patients' rights. In anticipation, Ohio ACEP provided data from Texas and Florida to legislators, demonstrating that similar bills improved access to care and did not increase complaints to state medical boards in those states. Furthermore, Ohio ACEP worked with the chair of the Senate committee to ensure the proceedings focused on evidence-based arguments, rather than on solely anecdotal stories designed to elicit emotional responses.[11]

Adversity and Regrouping

SB 86 passed through the Ohio Senate but was voted down in the House of Representatives in 2009-2010. Ohio ACEP worked to reintroduce the bill one year later as *SB 129*, following the 2010 state elections. The organization anticipated gaining the support of several new legislators and the new governor, whom they had helped elect to office. Ohio ACEP also faced unexpected challenges, however; one of SB 86's chief sponsors was promoted to the governor's office, depriving SB 129 of a key champion in the Senate. The newly elected Senate committee chair was less receptive to the language of the bill, and the opposition changed its strategy by producing an emergency physician to testify against it, arguing that the bill would foster the dangerous practice of medicine and decrease the access to quality care. These challenges continue to be addressed; the bill remains in the Senate committee.[11]

CONCLUSION

State-level advocacy, much like federal-level advocacy, is about building relationships, identifying supporters, and working toward a common goal. Many important issues for emergency medicine, including medical liability, health care reform implementation and challenges related to boarding and crowding, are best addressed on the state level. State politics may be smaller in terms of geography, but the advocacy approach is often the same. In fact, state and local lawmakers are much more accessible and willing to talk than their national counterparts, making advocacy much less daunting. If you are passionate about an issue, get involved and become an advocate! ✶

Additional Resources

- White House: www.whitehouse.gov/our-government/state-and-local-government
- National Conference of State Legislators: www.ncsl.org

Chapter **24**

HEALTH SERVICES RESEARCH

Brandon Maughan, MD, MHS

The science and sophistication of emergency medicine practice have been revolutionized over the last 30 years. Despite these improvements, many basic questions remain about how to most effectively deliver care to ED patients. Health services research (HSR) examines a wide range of topics that impact the organization, delivery, and financing of health care, many of which are pertinent to emergency medicine. HSR seeks to answer a variety of important questions, including:

- What percentage of of ED patients have primary care physicians? What fraction is uninsured?
- Which patients need imaging? How does imaging impact patient length of stay?
- How common is ED boarding and does it affect patient outcomes?
- How does ED communication with primary care providers impact patient outcomes? What is the best way to improve communication between these providers?
- Which parts of the country have the most effective trauma care systems? Do different types of EMS systems have different patient outcomes?
- What factors predict a patient's return to the ED within 72 hours?

Just as effective medical care is based on a foundation of clinical and translational research, health policy advocates rely on *health services* research to help define the problems facing our system and identify more effective ways to organize and pay for health care. HSR can measure the successes and failures of past health policy interventions and provide guidance on future policy design.

OVERVIEW OF HSR

Health services research has been defined in many different ways. In 2002, the Agency for Healthcare Research and Quality (AHRQ) described health services research as an examination of "how people get access to health care, how much care costs, and what happens to patients as a result of this care." AHRQ defined the primary goals of HSR as the identification of "the most effective ways to organize, manage, finance, and deliver high quality care; reduce medical errors; and improve patient safety."[1]

In contrast to basic science or clinical research that is focused on a single disease process or type of therapeutic intervention, HSR broadly examines public health, the structure of the health care system, the cost and quality of health care services, and ability (or inability) of populations to receive those services. Applications of HSR may range from a single emergency department to a large hospital system to the entire national health care system.

CHALLENGES IN STUDY DESIGN

Study designs and methods of analysis in HSR often differ from those used in clinical or translational research. Prospective study design and data collection often are regarded as necessary for the highest-quality clinical research; but, due to logistical challenges, they are uncommon in most HSR applications.

The *RAND Health Insurance Experiment* is a classic example of a health services study.[2] In this 15-year analysis, individuals were randomized to one of several different types of insurance, and researchers examined how this assignment affected their use of health care services. This landmark study collected data prospectively, but doing so required a multimillion dollar investment. Since prospective studies (including randomized controlled trials) often are logically infeasible, health services researchers use sophisticated statistical tools in their studies – including propensity scores, instrumental variables, multiple imputation, and adaptive trial design[3] – to account for confounders and missing data.

DATA SOURCES

Health services researchers often utilize large administrative databases or surveys to study state or nationwide trends. For example, the Centers for Disease Control and Prevention (CDC) manage the *National Hospital Ambulatory Medical Care Survey* (NHAMCS), an annual probability sample of visits to nonfederal hospital emergency departments and outpatient offices. NHAMCS collects a wide range of data, including (but not limited to) patient demographics, type of ED care providers, vital signs, diagnostic tests, medications, and diagnoses. This breadth of data collection allows researchers to address many different research questions without making the investments required by the RAND study.

In a recent study, researchers used NHAMCS data to measure how ED patients' lengths of stay were extended if they underwent blood tests, CT scan, or ultrasound. These results may help researchers project how changes in diagnostic imaging rates could impact patient flow and wait times.[4]

Using the same database, other investigators measured the utilization of midlevel providers in U.S. emergency departments from 2006 to 2009. They found that 5.8% of ED patients were seen by midlevel providers *without* physician involvement, and midlevel caregivers who worked in *rural* EDs saw a higher proportion of patients than those in *urban* EDs. These findings may motivate researchers to examine differences in cost and quality among physician and midlevel staffing in rural emergency departments.[5]

An analysis of NHAMCS data from 2001 to 2008, which studied the growth of observation care in U.S. emergency departments, found that the number of ED patients with dispositions to observation units increased nearly four-fold during the study period. This trend may guide future research on measuring the quality and cost-effectiveness of observation units.[6]

NHAMCS is not the only major database used by health services researchers. The Agency for Healthcare Research and Quality sponsors the *Healthcare Cost and Utilization Project* (HCUP), a set of several patient-level databases compiled in partnership with federal agencies, state governments, hospital associations, and private industry. HCUP databases that focus on emergency departments include the *National Emergency Department Sample* (NEDS) and *State Emergency Department Databases* (SEDD). Many other databases exist for specific questions in other research fields.

In addition to state and federal governments, nonprofit organizations play a major role in health services research. Examples of these organizations include *AcademyHealth*, the *Robert Wood Johnson Foundation*, the *Commonwealth Fund*, and the *Kaiser Family Foundation*. Many of these organizations have their own surveys and databases to guide policy research.

COMPARATIVE EFFECTIVENESS RESEARCH

Comparative effectiveness research (CER) is one type of HSR that examines the relative benefits, harms, and efficiency of different approaches to disease prevention, diagnosis, and treatment. In the 2009 American Recovery and Reinvestment Act (ARRA), Congress allocated $1.1 billion to promote the development of comparative effectiveness research. Whereas clinical trials often seek to identify the effectiveness of specific interventions in an idealized setting (e.g., assuming full patient compliance; excluding patients with certain comorbidities, without considering cost), CER seeks to identify how well these approaches work in real world settings and with consideration of costs.

Comparative effectiveness research historically has been more popular in countries outside the U.S., in which the government has a greater level of control over the health care system. The United Kingdom, for example, employs the *National Institute for Health and Clinical Excellence* (NICE), a division of the *English National Health Service* (NHS). The organization publishes evidence-based guidelines on "the most effective ways to diagnose, treat and prevent disease and ill health," based on evaluations of the efficacy and cost-effectiveness of various interventions and technologies. The recommendations of NICE guide the availability of treatment for patients utilizing the country's public health care system.

The Patient Protection and Affordable Care Act of 2010 established the Patient-Centered Outcomes Research Institute (PCORI). PCORI is an independent, nongovernmental organization whose mission is to develop CER that helps inform decision-making by both patients and health care providers. In particular, this research aims to integrate individual patient preferences regarding goals of treatment, including symptoms, mortality, and health-related quality of life.

IMPLICATIONS FOR ADVOCACY

In the coming years, high-quality comparative effectiveness research ideally will give physicians and patients the information necessary to make better-informed decisions about the cost, quality, and expected outcomes of different diagnostic and treatment options. Policymakers will use CER to influence cost-efficient medical decision-making, likely through a combination of publicly reported quality metrics and payment structure reforms.

Recent experience with proposed CMS quality measure OP-15, which measured emergency department use of CT scans for atraumatic headaches, demonstrates that these quality measures must be designed very carefully. Emergency medicine advocates armed with evidence from HSR can help shape the appropriate development of these measures, as they have with OP-15.

CONCLUSION

Health services research will continue to guide the development, evaluation, and reform of health policy on state, federal, and international levels. In an era of increasing focus on health care cost and efficiency, a generation of new health services researchers in emergency medicine will help revolutionize the way health care is delivered.

With recent federal investments in CER, researchers soon will have the tools to better analyze the relative costs, benefits, and risks associated with diagnostic and treatment decisions. As with any area of new research, initial research may be limited in scope, but the role of CER will grow as patients and physicians embrace its application. ✴

Chapter 25

MEDICAL LIABILITY REFORM

Brian Kloss, DO, JD, PA-C

Medical liability reform, previously referred to as "tort reform," has been a recurrent challenge over the last 50 years through the multiple crises in medical malpractice coverage. A *tort* is a civil law proceeding in which an injured party seeks compensation, usually monetary, for the harm they suffered at the hands of another. *Medical liability reform* generally refers to legislative proposals to limit or regulate legal claims brought to court that are perceived to unfairly burden defendants and insurance policy holders. In laymen's terms, medical liability reform tends to deal more specifically with reforming *medical malpractice* litigation. Although medical liability reform traditionally has been a matter of state common law and legislation, the issue has become a more prominent focus of federal legislators.

WHAT IS THE "MALPRACTICE CRISIS"?

There have been three major malpractice crises in modern times; each is defined by a substantial increase in premium rates, a decrease in the number of insurers offering malpractice coverage, and a deterioration of the financial health of the insurance companies. These phenomena lead to changes in physician practice decisions and decreased provider availability. As various states and government entities increasingly have been under pressure from their constituents to address these issues, there have been incremental changes in some state laws.

In the 1970s, the malpractice crisis was one of insurance *availability*. With insurers leaving volatile markets, physicians were unable to find coverage, regardless of price.[1] This led to successful liability reform campaigns in a few states, including California, which enacted the prototypical medical liability reform model, the Medical Injury Compensation Reform Act (MIRCA) of 1975.[2] MIRCA placed a $250,000 cap on non-economic damages, set regulations on attorney contingency fees, and altered the collateral source rule, thus allowing juries to be informed of other potentially responsible parties who may already have compensated the plaintiff.[3]

In the 1980s, another surge of premium increases swept across the country, leading to a crisis of insurance *affordability*. In response, physicians cut back on both high-risk procedures and high-risk patients; and, in some instances, physicians opted to close their practices entirely. Many physicians turned to local joint underwriting associations for liability coverage, despite the high cost, while others opted to "go bare" and practice medicine without *any* malpractice insurance coverage.

The third major crisis developed at the turn of the 21st century. Concerns have persisted about continued litigation, which ultimately have translated into a decrease in access to insurance markets. Physician response to concerns over increasing malpractice premiums and decreasing reimbursements has led some high-risk physicians to narrow their scopes of practice, opt for early retirement, and/or change practice locations. The overall effect has meant that patients must travel further for care, change physicians, and wait longer for emergency and surgical treatment.[4]

WHAT ARE PHYSICIANS' CONCERNS?

There is a general concern among many physicians that the current system encourages lawsuits through excessive payouts in a lottery-like system. In one study, 74% of malpractice claims closed without payment,[5] of which 37% did not involve a medical error and 3% did not involve a patient injury.[6] Ironically, despite arguments that lawsuits reduce the rates of patient injury and act as a "checks and balances" toward quality patient care, concern exists that the litigious atmosphere may shift physician practices from evidenced-based to *defensive* medicine. As a result, patients may be exposed to unnecessary tests and the associated risks and costs; or, in the other extreme, patients who may benefit from riskier procedures may have care withheld for fear of a bad outcome resulting in a lawsuit.

The issue of defensive medicine increasingly is being examined as a source of significant cost to the U.S. health care system. In one study, 93% of high-risk specialty physicians reported practicing defensive medicine and admitted that behaviors such as ordering unnecessary lab tests or imaging studies, requesting specialty consultations, and referring patients to other providers were "very common" in their practices.[7] In addition, 42% of respondents took steps to restrict their practices, including the elimination of high-risk scenarios prone to complications (trauma surgery, for example; or caring for patients with complex medical histories or those perceived as litigious).[7] Physicians, patients, and employers bear the brunt of excessive litigation; the direct and indirect costs of malpractice claims are recouped through increased premiums and the cost of medical care. The *exact* cost to the health care system is controversial, however. While the Congressional Budget Office estimates the added cost at $54 billion over 10 years,[13] other sources estimate costs that are orders of magnitude higher, from $55.6 billion annually[14] to as high as $850 billion a year.[15]

WHAT IS THE SOLUTION?

The number of proposals that have been developed is extensive. To effectively advocate for change, it is imperative to understand the issues and proposed solutions. Options include:[8,10]

- **Caps on Non-economic Damages.** *Economic* damages represent the loss of quantifiable income due to injury or death, including personal income, medical costs, and future care costs. These are quantifiable costs, based on an individual's previous function and/or potential before the injury, and are relatively limited in comparison to non-economic or punitive damages.

Non-economic damages are those that cannot necessarily be quantified, such as suffering, consortium (e.g., companionship and sexual intimacy) and vision. Punitive damages serve as a means of enacting economic punishment against the defendant for his or her wrongdoing. Legislative action to cap non-economic damages, more recently a discussion on the federal level, traditionally has been regulated by individual states. According to the American Tort Reform Association, 37 states have enacted legislation that limits non-economic damages.[3] In many states, these caps are being challenged as unconstitutional; laws enacting economic caps have been overturned in at least 11 states, whereas similar laws in at least 16 other states have been upheld. Most recently, the cap on non-economic damages was upheld in the state of Kansas in 2012, while a similar cap was found unconstitutional two months earlier in Missouri.

- **Joint and Several Liability Reform.** Forty states have enacted reform for a proportionate liability system, where each co-defendant is liable for his or her proportion of harm to the plaintiff. As a result, individual defendants are required to pay no more than their share of the damages awarded to the plaintiff.[11] Let's say, for example, that a jury awards a plaintiff $2 million. If the emergency medicine physician is found to be 10% at fault and a neurosurgeon is found to be 90% at fault, the emergency medicine physician (or his liability insurer) would be required to pay only $200,000 (10% of the damages). Prior to these reforms, each individual defendant could be held 100% liable for damages, regardless of individually assessed liability. Without this type of reform, plaintiff attorneys were more inclined to name defendants who had "big pockets," not necessarily those who were at fault for the care in question.

- **Comparative Negligence Reform.** Similar to joint and several liability, in which a plaintiff is held partially responsible for his own injury, the award could be reduced by a proportional amount. For example, if a patient undergoes a complicated knee repair surgery and is non-complaint with the surgeon's post-operative recommendations and physical therapy appointments, and the knee subsequently becomes damaged, the plaintiff can be found partially responsible due to his lack of adherence to physician recommendations. Without any consideration of comparative negligence, the orthopedic surgeon could still be considered 100% liable for damages.

- **Collateral Source Rule Reform.** In states without this reform, evidence may not be admitted at trial to show if – or how much – of the plaintiff's losses have already been compensated from other sources, including insurance or worker's compensation. As a result, a plaintiff can "double-dip" and, in some instances, collect twice or more for the same injury. As an example: A postal worker slips and falls outside of an individual's house on a snowy day, requiring emergent orthopedic surgery that results in a poor outcome. The postal worker can collect workman's compensation from his employer, can collect monies from the homeowner's insurance policy where the injury occurred, and can file a suit against the orthopedic surgeon. Economic damages, such as medical bills and lost wages, can be collected from *all three parties* for the *same* injury. Twenty-four states have enacted legislation that has reformed this rule.[11]

- **Limitation on Attorney's Fees.** One of the most contested reforms has been the implementation of *caps* or controls on attorney fees and compensation. As it stands, most personal injury and malpractice cases operate on a contingency basis. There are no costs for the plaintiff if the attorney fails to settle or win the case. Attorney contingency fees can range from one-third to one-half of the monetary award, but are not calculated until overhead expenses have been paid out. Reform proposals seek to put more money in the hands of the injured party, and not the attorney who worked the case. These reforms target high-cost cases in which a 30-40% contingency fee may lead to *millions* in attorney compensation. Many argue the current system encourages a lottery-like mentality that leads attorneys to take cases with little merit, in hope of getting a favorable jury at trial.

- **Qualification for Expert Witnesses.** Under traditional evidentiary standards, a witness may be an "expert" if he or she has the education, training, or experience to testify about issues in a case. Reform measures in some states have included clinical duty requirements, similar practice backgrounds, board certification, or actual professional knowledge based on active practice. In states without reform to this rule, a retired clinical neurologist who has neither seen nor treated a patient in more than 15 years could serve as the "expert" witness against an emergency medicine physician. In a setting *with* reform, the court standard would require an emergency medicine physician of similar training and experience (and still active in clinical practice) to serve as the expert witness.

- **Statutes of Limitation/Response Reform.** Statutes of limitation place constraints on the time in which a lawsuit can be filed. The clock starts ticking at either the time the incident allegedly occurred or the date that the malpractice was discovered (termed the "discovery rule"). The *statute of repose* provides an absolute limit on time, regardless of the discovery rule, allowing for the risk to end a definitive point in time. Many states do not have such a statute. Other reforms have proposed shortening the time to suit, especially in the setting of pediatric cases that last until the child reaches the age of majority (typically, age 18). In states without a statute of repose or limitation in the case of minors, obstetrical and pediatric insurance can be very expensive due to the long tail coverage required.

- **Specialized Health Courts.** Specialized courts could be developed to deal specifically with issues of medical malpractice, and specially trained attorneys would handle these cases. Similar courts currently exist in the United States to deal with issues of tax and maritime law. Proponents argue that such a reform would expedite the judicial process and provide more consistent outcomes for plaintiffs. However, such change would likely require a Constitutional amendment; the Seventh Amendment currently permits all suits at common law, in excess of $20, to preserve the right to a trial by jury.[12] States such as Utah have enacted health courts by creating an advisory panel prior to trial; if a party disregards the findings, it is exposed to attorney's fees from the opposing party.

- **Loser Pays.** One of the more extreme proposals of medical liability reforms suggests the adoption of the British system, wherein the court costs and legal fees of the prevailing party are paid for by the party that lost the suit. Proponents advocate that such a change would limit the number of frivolous lawsuits, while opponents are concerned that such policies would have a chilling effect on plaintiff's rights to file claims for compensation.

- **No-Fault System.** As the name implies, *no fault* is assigned to either party and claims are paid to recipients of poor medical care from a collective insurance pool, possibly governmentally administered. This type of system would reduce litigation costs, put money into the injured party's hands more quickly, and would better regulate and standardize compensation. A similar model currently exists for workmen's compensation and disability.

- **Extend FTCA Coverage.** Under EMTALA, emergency medicine practitioners are required to provide examination and stabilization to all patients presenting to an emergency department, regardless of their abilities to pay. The Federal Tort Claims Act limits the liability of individual practitioners and requires that a plaintiff file suit against the federal government when a defendant was acting under his or her scope of practice. Extending FTCA coverage to care provided under EMTALA would decrease the liability incurred by emergency physicians and consulting specialists when providing emergency care, which is frequently uncompensated. The FTCA currently covers medical liability for employees at federally supported health centers and free clinics, as well as federally owned systems such as the Veterans Affairs system and the Indian Health Service.

DEMONSTRATION PROJECTS

The ACA authorizes up to $50 million in grants for the Department of Health and Human Services (HHS) to award to states for the planning of demonstration projects to develop, implement, and evaluate alternatives to the current medical malpractice litigation system in the next five years. Potential reforms could include developing health courts or requiring that medical liability cases be reviewed by independent physicians prior to trial. The secretary of HHS can grant an applicant state an initial $500,000 as a planning grant for the development of demonstration project applications. However, these grants come with many requirements, including the caveat that participants must be voluntary and maintain the right to withdraw from the program at any time. While funds for this program were scheduled to be available beginning in 2011, the administration had not made any requests to fund the program at press time and Congress had not appropriated any dollars for it.

STATES AS LABORATORIES

While there has been little recent federal action on liability reform, states have continued to look for ways to improve their medical liability systems. Texas recently became the "poster child" for state-based reform. During the 78th Legislature in 2003, the Texas statehouse passed comprehensive tort reform, including limits on non-economic damages. The intention was to address the increasing health care costs precipitated by the practice of defensive medicine by reducing the number of lawsuits being brought against physicians and medical groups. The effect of this legislation has been mixed. Current data shows that the number of medical liability lawsuits has decreased and that more physicians are being drawn to the state, improving access to care; however, health care costs have not fallen significantly as a result of the reforms. Many other states are still considering or implementing caps, although their constitutionality continues to be questioned.

CONCLUSION

Emergency physicians are high-risk specialists who care for some of the sickest patients in health care, without regard to their abilities to pay. We provide this care emergently, without the luxuries of pre-existing relationships with our patients or complete access to their medical histories. Providing liability protection to physicians for the federally-mandated EMTALA services we provide will help ensure emergency and on-call physicians remain available to treat patients in their communities. To control costs and protect our patients and ourselves, we must fix the broken system by continuing to advocate for reforms that honor quality care. ✳

Chapter 26

CORPORATE PRACTICE OF MEDICINE

Sarah Hoper, MD, JD

The issue of *corporate medicine* has been a part of health care for more than 150 years. It remains a topic of controversy today, as the nation demands the medical industry cut costs and adopt business management models. Some believe that by allowing lay corporations to operate clinics and physician groups, physicians will lose their autonomy and develop divided loyalties between their patients and their employer. There are more corporate medicine jobs for emergency physicians every year, however, and the health care industry increasingly is using lay-owned groups in other medical specialties. With 50% of physicians now employed by hospitals or other health care entities, the implications of the corporate practice and the need for physician autonomy in patient care is of critical importance.[1]

HISTORY

The *corporate practice of medicine doctrine* was conceived by the American Medical Association (AMA) in 1847. During that time, physicians were having difficulty distinguishing themselves from "irregulars." *Irregulars* were described as faith healers, people selling door-to-door elixirs, and others without traditional medical training.[2] The AMA adopted the *Code of 1847*, which prohibited physicians from engaging in entrepreneurial activities, such as holding patents on medicine or instruments, promoting secret remedies and advertising to enhance their own reputations.[3]

> *Many hospitals are nonprofit organizations and are presumed to lack a profit motive; therefore, the physician cannot be torn between the hospital's goals and what is best for his patients. In states that do not have laws that apply specifically to hospitals, the courts have been lax in their interpretation of corporate practice of medicine laws or have created specific exceptions for hospitals.*

In the early twentieth century, three new business models arose. The first was *contract practice*, whereby a company would hire a physician to take care of its employees and their families. The second was *corporate practice*, in which corporations hired physicians and marketed them to the general public. The third format was the inception of the hospital. The AMA feared these business models were threats to physician autonomy, patient load, methods of treatment and diagnosis, and would lead to the loss of the physician's control over his own income. The AMA then sought to establish the autonomy of physicians as independent decision-makers, who cared only for the *scientific* treatment of patients. The AMA insisted on the licensing of medical doctors, deeming them the sole legitimate providers of health care.[4]

DEFINITION OF CORPORATE PRACTICE OF MEDICINE

Today, the corporate practice of medicine doctrine prohibits unlicensed individuals and corporations from engaging in the practice of medicine by restricting them from employing licensed physicians. The intent of the doctrine is to ensure that physicians' medical decisions are not influenced by their employers' business objectives. Based on this doctrine, 30 states have enacted laws that ban lay persons and corporations from employing physicians to practice medicine.[5] This restricts the delivery of medical services to those corporations and limited liability partnerships that are solely owned by licensed physicians and whose shareholders are all licensed physicians.

These entities are called *professional corporations* (PC). The law allows physicians to be independent contractors for lay corporations because the physician presumably retains autonomy over professional decisions and has no duty of loyalty owed to the employer. The corporate practice of medicine doctrine also prohibits fee-splitting between licensed physicians and lay individuals or corporations.[6] Many states also have legislation that bans fee splitting.

HMOs often are lay-owned corporations, but they are governed under a separate set of federal laws. Under preemption principles, federal law *replaces* state law where there is a conflict. Consequently, states must provide an exception to existing corporate practice bans and allow lay-owned HMOs to hire physicians. In many states, hospitals also are governed under separate laws, allowing hospitals to directly employ physicians rather than hiring them as independent contractors.

Many hospitals are nonprofit organizations and are presumed to lack a profit motive; therefore, the physician cannot be torn between the hospital's goals and what is best for his patients. In states that do not have laws that apply specifically to hospitals, the courts have been lax in their interpretation of corporate practice of medicine laws or have created specific exceptions for hospitals.[7] As such, legislation outlawing the corporate practice of medicine primarily applies to outpatient clinics and staffing entities known as *physician practice management companies* (PPMC), which supply physicians to certain practice environments, including emergency departments.

PHYSICIAN PRACTICE MANAGEMENT COMPANIES[8]

PPMCs are lay-owned companies that provide management services consisting of billing, the provision of capital for practice development, contract negotiation, office space and equipment, insurance, accounting, legal services, and other non-professional personnel services.

In states with laws prohibiting the corporate practice of medicine, PPMCs often get around the law by setting up professional corporations (PC) that provide management services for the company. The PC's stock is owned entirely by a small number of physicians who are contractually bound to the lay-owned PPMC. The stockholders will then hire the physicians needed to staff a clinic or emergency department. The professional corporation is bound by the agreement with the physician management company to enforce the contract requirements. These mandates may include productivity standards, hiring requirements for providers, compensation and the provision of incentive packages (often designed by the PPMC), and general compliance with the PPMC's management agreement. The PC will own all of the revenue from the practice, but the PC will be required to pay a percentage of the revenue to the PPMC. In states with laws against fee-splitting, the professional corporation may pay a flat rate for administrative services to the PPMC.

DEFINITION OF FEE-SPLITTING

Historically, a physician engaged in illegal fee-splitting by dividing a patient's fee with a referring physician. Today, many states have laws that do not allow physicians to share a percentage of their medical professional fees with anyone other than the physicians with whom they practice. In these states, physicians are prohibited from making percentage-of-profit payments for any purpose, including payments to PPMCs, which may have built-in incentives to overbill. In many states that prohibit fee-splitting, however, physicians can pay a flat fee for those services. Interestingly, some states that ban physician fee-splitting *allow* the division of payments generated by nurse practitioners, physician assistants, and physical therapists; the services granted by these providers are not defined as *professional medical services*. Some states do not have *any* laws against fee splitting.

INFLUENCE OF PROFIT, AUTONOMY AND QUALITY OF HEALTH CARE

Recent cases on the corporate practice of medicine have focused on the influence of profit, the loss of the physician's autonomy, and the quality of health care. The motive for profit exists in all professions and in all types of health care arrangements, including independent contract relationships, professional corporations, nonprofit organizations, and PPMCs. Physicians and professional corporations cannot enter into independent contracts that are not sustainable, as evidenced by the increasing number of physicians refusing to take Medicare and Medicaid patients.

Likewise, nonprofit organizations are acutely aware of the amount of revenue needed to continue to grow their institutions and can exert pressure on their employees to produce the needed funds. The *Institute of Medicine* acknowledges that all current payment methods are likely to affect behavior, and argues that payment incentives should be based on the quality of medicine provided and quality improvement, thereby using profit motivation to the benefit of the patient.[9] This is the current strategy employed by CMS and other payers regarding *value-based purchasing, never events* and other quality-driven payment decisions.

Loss of physician autonomy is another concern in any employment arrangement. There is a persistent fear that physicians will lose their ability to decide which and how many patients to see, and how to treat their patients. Many believe that the loss of autonomy, as well as the drive for profits, will lead to a decrease in the quality of health care provided to patients. Employers will demand that physicians see more patients in order to increase profit margins at the expense of good medical care. Yet, with HMOs, we already have accepted the risk of lay control in favor of the efficiency that accompanies managed health care. Federal and many states' HMO regulations assert that business arrangements may not interfere with the independent professional judgment of physicians, thereby hoping to protect physician autonomy.[10]

Similarly, there are increasing numbers of accountable care organizations; as of November 2012, there were 328 CMS-recognized ACOs serving 2.4 million Medicare patients and 15 million non-Medicare patients.[11] ACOs also have been granted exceptions to the laws regarding the corporate practice of medicine. Physicians will continue to be subject to professional ethical standards and licensing statutes that will also help protect against lay interference in the practice of medicine.

CONCLUSION

Despite concerns about the loss of physician autonomy, the influence of profit, and the quality of health care, HMOs, teaching hospitals, nonprofit hospitals and other lay-owned organizations have become an accepted part of our health care system. HMOs, PPOs, PPMCs, and now ACOs, also are being heavily relied upon to help control health care costs. With the acceptance of other lay-owned health organizations and an increasing need to curb costs, it may be unreasonable to single out PPMCs as violators of the corporate practice of medicine.

Most importantly, every emergency physician must be aware of the details of his or her contract – whether it is with a hospital, PC, HMO, ACO or PPMC. A physician must know whether his or her contract has an "open book" policy or includes a non-compete clause; and must understand the type of malpractice insurance the employer will provide (whether it is *claims made, occurrence coverage,* or *claims paid*), and how that will affect the physician's ability to leave a new job. It also is critical to understand if a contract is "at will" (meaning that either party can terminate the employment at any time without cause); physicians must demand better contracts when confronted with unfair terms. ✶

Chapter 27

REGIONALIZATION

K Kay Moody, DO, MPH and Alison Haddock, MD

Regionalization in the United States began with regionalization of trauma care and has subsequently expanded to include additional diagnoses, particularly stroke and ST-elevation myocardial infarction. The move toward regionalization of emergency services developed in response to numerous factors, including lack of specialist coverage in rural areas and documented improved patient outcomes in high-volume specialty settings. Conditions for which timely delivery of specialized treatment (such as emergency trauma surgery, percutaneous coronary intervention, or lytic administration) can be lifesaving and are particularly amenable to regionalization.

The basic idea of "regionalizing" care involves bypassing the closest hospital to transport a patient to a specialty center in the area of care required by the patient. The principle can be controversial, as some report improved patient outcomes at large centers, but others advocate for more localized and potentially faster availability of potentially lifesaving care.

Treatment of the acutely injured patient is integral to the core mission of emergency medicine; injuries are the number one cause of death for Americans under the age of 45, making this care critically important.[1] The development of trauma systems to optimize care for these patients has been ongoing during the past 50 years, but progress has been slow and uneven. It serves as a case study for the role of political action in the development of our health care system and may be a model for future regionalization of medical emergency care.

Regionalization is a broad term. The basic idea of "regionalizing" care involves bypassing the closest hospital to transport a patient to a specialty center in the area of triage required by the patient. The principle can be controversial, as some report improved patient outcomes at large centers, but others advocate for more localized and potentially faster availability of potentially lifesaving care.

Those in favor of regionalization report evidence of decreased morbidity and mortality for patients who receive their care from a designated center that manages a great number of cases of STEMI, stroke, or trauma and is equipped with specialized staff and supplies. Some worry, however, that regionalization may disenfranchise small rural hospitals, which may not have an adequate volume of cases or enough financial resources to establish and maintain accreditation. Lack of accreditation may also prevent these hospitals from serving as residency training sites, potentially further limiting the availability of emergency physicians in non-urban regions.

TRAUMA CENTERS

The *trauma system* concept developed from the military experience of WWI and WWII, as injured soldiers were taken from the battlefield to an emergency care station, then to a hospital for definitive surgical management.[2] In the first half of the 20th century, urban hospitals began to imitate this model with systems of pre-hospital care and patient transfer; yet, no states had a formal trauma system in place.

Government leadership in trauma care began with the 1966 publication of "Accidental Death and Disability: The Neglected Disease of Modern Society" by the National Academy of Sciences (NAS).[3] This manuscript emphasized the large burden of accidental death and injury on society and included a set of wide-ranging recommendations, calling upon the public and the government to improve pre-hospital care by setting standards for ambulance services, improve research into accident prevention and trauma care, and develop trauma registries and committees. Most importantly, the NAS recommended "programs to establish patterns of and numbers and types of emergency departments necessary for optimal care of emergency surgical and medical casualties" and the "development of a mechanism for inspection, categorization and accreditation of emergency rooms on a continuing basis."[3]

The report was followed by the passage of the *National Highway Safety Act of 1966*, in which Congress provided funding to improve motor vehicle safety and the care of injured patients. Money was specifically earmarked to encourage the development of effective regional emergency services programs, including trauma systems. Maryland and Illinois were early leaders in the field and created two of the first regionalized trauma systems in the country, establishing Shock Trauma in Baltimore in 1969[2] and Cook County Hospital in Chicago in 1971.[4] Research conducted after the creation of these systems suggests that the changes significantly decreased mortality for critically injured trauma patients. These findings bolstered public and professional support for nationwide creation of trauma systems.

Despite this evidence of improved outcomes, trauma system development in many states floundered. Further progress remained dependent on money. When federal funds were widely available in the 1970s, states responded by creating 304 EMS regions across the United States by 1978; but as funding declined (as in 1981, when the Omnibus Budget Reconciliation Act eliminated federal funding for EMS), progress slowed. In the absence of national governmental support, leadership from organized medicine and public advocacy became increasingly important.

The American College of Surgeons (ACS) stepped into trauma system development in 1976, when the Committee on Trauma (COT) released its first edition of *Optimal Hospital Resources for the Care of the Seriously Injured*. This manual is regularly revised[5] and continues to set the standard for necessary trauma center resources. The ACS developed a voluntary process in which hospitals may undergo review by the *COT Verification Committee* and be named an "ACS-Verified" Level I or Level II Trauma Center. In its publications, the ACS emphasizes the importance of regional trauma systems to improve outcomes.

Despite these efforts, many states remained without fully implemented trauma systems throughout the 1970s and 1980s. In 1990, federal funding for trauma regionalization was reestablished with the passage of the *Trauma Care Systems Planning and Development Act*.[2] Federal funds were provided for trauma systems, but states balked as they found the federal model to be excessively restrictive; funding for the act was not reauthorized in 1995, so its long-term impact has been limited.

A national survey of trauma systems in 1993[6] found that 20 states had a formal process for the designation of trauma centers, using at least some of the ACS criteria. Only five of these states, however, met a complete set of criteria defining an effective trauma system. These criteria included statewide trauma center coverage; a method for ongoing monitoring of the system; and crucially, limitations on the number of trauma centers based on population need. Limiting designated trauma centers is politically challenging, as hospitals and neighborhoods are eager to earn the designation. At the core of any trauma system, however, is the principle that the concentration of the most severely injured patients will increase patient volume and experience at these centers, thus improving patient outcomes and controlling costs by preventing the unnecessary duplication of expensive resources.

Ongoing evidence supports the assertion that regionalization of trauma care improves outcomes. One large study recently examined the effect of care at a Level I trauma center on risk of death in adult patients with moderate to severe traumatic injury; it found that the risk of death within one year after injury was significantly lower when care was provided in a trauma center.[7] Another study compared data from all 50 states and concluded that those states with trauma systems in place for at least 10 years experienced an 8% reduction in mortality from motor vehicle collisions.[8]

Unfortunately, this compelling collection of evidence has not led to universal adoption of statewide trauma regionalization. The most recent comprehensive review of trauma centers[9] found that, as of April 2002, only 35 states and the District of Columbia had formally designated and certified trauma centers. While this is an increase from the 20 states with systems at the time of the 1993 review, there persists a lack of comprehensive trauma regionalization in the United States. The number of trauma centers doubled between 1991 and 2002, but coverage of rural areas in many states remains sparse. In addition, many trauma centers in urban areas face intermittent budget crises due to poor reimbursement for the care they deliver to indigent patients, particularly those with severe penetrating injuries in high-crime areas.

STROKE CENTERS

Following the model of trauma, experts in neurology and emergency medicine have initiated regionalization for stroke care. Their efforts began after it was established that timely delivery of tissue plasminogen activator (tPA) could reduce morbidity and mortality in stroke, and the drug was approved by the FDA.[10] A multidisciplinary group of representatives from major professional organizations formed, calling themselves the "Brain Attack Coalition." This group authored a paper in 2000,[11] outlining the essential care needed for patients suffering from acute stroke. Key elements included acute stroke teams, stroke units, written care protocols, and an integrated emergency response system, as well as 24-hour rapid availability of computer tomography scans and laboratory testing. Hospitals with these capabilities are designated as *Primary Stroke Centers*.

In December 2003, the Joint Commission launched a program to certify hospitals that incorporate all of these elements into the care they deliver to stroke patients[12]. The certification process is voluntary, and is intended to help hospitals ensure that they are providing high-quality care. As part of the certification and recertification process, the Joint Commission requires that certified centers track and report on eight quality measures specific to stroke care (see Table).

Core Measures for Primary Stroke Centers[12]

•	Venous thromboembolism (VTE) prophylaxis
•	Discharged on antithrombotic therapy
•	Anticoagulation therapy for atrial fibrillation/flutter
•	Thrombolytic therapy
•	Antithrombotic therapy by end of hospital day two
•	Discharged on statin medication
•	Stroke education
•	Assessed for rehabilitation

Many states have established policies that define Primary Stroke Centers.[13] In most cases, this has come in the form of legislation; however, statewide administrative policies, including executive orders and administrative rules, also have been utilized by a number of states. While a few of these states have hospital bypass policies (directing EMS to deliver stroke patients only to certified stroke centers), most states focus on educating EMS providers and encouraging EMS systems to develop protocols for the optimal management of patients with suspected stroke.[13] While small community hospitals may lobby for this approach in order to maintain their patient volumes, there is accumulating evidence that patient outcomes are improved when EMS delivers patients with suspected stroke directly to stroke centers.[10] The latest data showed that, in 2010, only 14 states had passed formal legislation to establish primary stroke centers.[13] As of 2012, there are more than 925 Joint Commission-certified primary stroke centers, with at least one in every state.[12,13]

The *Brain Attack Coalition* continued to work toward regionalization of stroke care by defining *comprehensive stroke centers* (CSC) in 2005.[14] In order to be classified as a CSC, hospitals were required to provide additional specialized components of care, including health care personnel with specific expertise in a number of disciplines (including neurosurgery and vascular neurology), advanced neuroimaging capabilities, surgical and endovascular techniques, and other specific infrastructure and programmatic elements, such as an intensive care unit and a stroke registry. The concept of a CSC was modeled after a Level 1 trauma center and is intended to allow patients with more advanced needs (such as those with large ischemic strokes or hemorrhagic strokes, those with strokes from unusual etiologies, those requiring specialized testing or therapies, or those requiring multispecialty management) to receive the most specialized care.[15]

The Joint Commission was slower to embrace the concept of comprehensive stroke centers, as the evidence for improved outcomes with the availability of additional resources (such as neurointerventional techniques) remains mixed. In 2012, however, the Joint Commission developed an *Advanced Certification for Comprehensive Stroke Centers;*[15] this development is a significant advance for regionalization in the field of stroke care, and has the potential to further improve outcomes for patients with complex disease processes.

> To further decrease the time from onset of myocardial infarction to PCI, improvements in patient education and EMS systems will be necessary. Patients persistently fail to recognize cardiac symptoms, and both delay seeking care and use personal transportation to arrive at the hospital in favor of calling 9-1-1.

Multiple studies have shown improved morbidity and mortality for stroke patients when they are cared for at a designated stroke center;[10] patients and providers must continue advocacy efforts on a state level to ensure that adults with acute stroke receive the fastest and highest quality care possible in their regions.

CARDIAC CARE

Much like trauma and stroke, an ST-elevation myocardial infarction (STEMI) is a defined disease process that shows significant improvements in morbidity and mortality when lifesaving treatment is rapidly delivered. While the efforts of the American College of Surgeons and the Brain Attack Coalition, among other organizations, have led to the establishment of standards to define both trauma and stroke centers, there is no nationally recognized program to define a *myocardial infarction center.*

It has long been acknowledged that the best treatment for STEMI is prompt percutaneous coronary intervention (PCI).[16] The Center for Medicare and Medicaid Services (CMS) and the Joint Commission have adopted "door to balloon time," as a core measure of hospital quality; shorter time from arrival in the ED to primary percutaneous intervention is proven to improve outcomes for STEMI patients. Of the more than 5,000 acute care hospitals in the U.S., however, only 1,176 are capable of performing PCI.[17]

While there have been calls for a nationwide system of regionalization to direct patients with STEMI to hospitals with PCI capabilities, regionalization instead has occurred on local and statewide levels. The latest data from the American Heart Association's *Mission: Lifeline* identified 381 unique systems involving 899 percutaneous coronary intervention hospitals in 47 states, creating a complex web of networks to direct patients to the nearest PCI-capable hospital.[18] Despite the complexities of this system, recent years have seen an improvement in door-to-balloon time for patients nationwide.[19]

Some large and well-coordinated systems have developed, including North Carolina's statewide *Regional Approach to Cardiovascular Emergencies* (RACE) project. Implementation of RACE resulted in improvement in door-to-device time, as well as a decrease in the number of patients not receiving reperfusion, and demonstrated that EMS-transported patients were most likely to reach door-to-device goals.[20] Further regionalization of STEMI care would benefit from more widespread adoption of standardized guidelines (such as the American Heart Association's criteria for the ideal system for the STEMI-receiving hospital[21]), as well as interventions to decrease delays in care for patients who are transferred to receive PCI.[22]

To further decrease the time from onset of myocardial infarction to PCI, improvements in patient education and EMS systems will be necessary. Patients persistently fail to recognize cardiac symptoms, and both delay seeking care and use personal transportation to arrive at the hospital in favor of calling 9-1-1. In a 2011 study, EMS transport was used for only 60% of patients with myocardial infarction.[23] To optimize care for patients who use EMS, pre-hospital EKGs must be performed and coupled with communication of STEMI diagnosis and preferential transport to a PCI-capable hospital, as this has been clearly demonstrated to speed time to reperfusion and improve clinical outcomes.[24] Interventions in these areas and improved coordination and systematic regionalization will decrease time to reperfusion and, consequently, decrease morbidity and mortality for the thousands of Americans experiencing acute myocardial infarctions each year.

FUTURE OF REGIONALIZATION

In a publication comparable to the 1966 National Academy of Sciences report on accidental injury, the Institute of Medicine published "Hospital Based Emergency Care: At The Breaking Point" in 2006. The report recommended establishment of a "regionalized, coordinated and accountable" system of emergency care. The goal of regionalized care is to ensure that emergency patients receive "the right care at the right place at the right time," but the best method for accomplishing that goal remains unclear.

On a national level, the *Emergency Care and Coordination Center* (ECCC) was established in 2009 within the Department of Health and Human Services; it aims to serve as a lead federal agency for accomplishing regionalization, but is still developing. Additionally, the ACA included a provision stating that funding would be made available to "support pilot projects that design, implement, and evaluate innovative models of regionalized, comprehensive, and accountable emergency care and trauma systems." This funding may be the crucial next step toward putting emergency medical care on the path to formalized regionalization on a state-by-state basis. In order to effectively execute this process, it is instructive to remember the challenges of trauma regionalization: limiting the number of specialty centers to maximize experience and decrease costs; adequately covering underserved areas; developing registries to monitor outcomes; and maintaining steady funding to maintain advances and prevent regression.

While nationwide legislation may provide an important source of funding, current efforts towards establishing regionalized networks of care primarily occur on a state-by-state level. In addition to current efforts regarding the care of patients with STEMI and stroke, other areas of interest include pediatric critical care and out-of-hospital cardiac arrest (to expedite therapeutic hypothermia). These efforts continue to face challenges prior to their implementation. Barriers include opposition from less specialized hospitals; concern about their abilities to compete if they cannot earn the special designations of regionalization; and the many challenges facing emergency medicine as a whole, including problems with crowding and diversion, fragmented care, inadequate disaster preparedness, limited emergency-focused research and workforce challenges.

CONCLUSION

In the past 50 years, trauma systems slowly have developed in most areas of the United States. Stroke centers are becoming well-established nationwide; STEMI centers remain a regional patchwork, but are increasingly effective at directing appropriate patients for prompt intervention at PCI-capable hospitals. Health services researchers have led the way to regionalization by highlighting the large burden of disease and the evidence that coordinated care can reduce morbidity and mortality; pioneering individuals have guided their states and institutions to create some of the first systems of regionalized trauma transport.

Financing from the federal government has been a key motivator for states to create and improve their systems. Additionally, organized medicine has played a role in setting standards for the certification and formal acknowledgement of trauma and stroke centers. In the wake of health care reform, researchers, governmental organizations, organized medicine, individual leaders, and emergency physicians must continue to apply the lessons of the past to create the best possible system of regionalized emergency medical care. *

Chapter 28

ETHICS IN ADVOCACY

Kael DuPrey, MD, JD

Ethics, or moral philosophy, is a branch of philosophy that involves defending, recommending and systematizing notions of right and wrong behavior.[1] The word itself means "character" in Greek (*ethos*). Ethics are fundamental to the advocacy and lobbying landscape and consist of various rules. The First Amendment states that the American people have a right "to petition the government for a redress of grievances"; the right to lobby and advocate for your cause is constitutionally protected. This chapter discusses ethics and how they relate to advocacy, and aims to enlighten your own advocacy efforts on the local, state or national levels.

PRIVACY CONCERNS

Situation/hypothetical. *You are a busy emergency medicine practitioner; you have done your homework and successfully arranged a meeting with your representative. One of the best ways to persuade is through an illustrative story about patient care in your emergency department. You want to describe a moving patient encounter you had. What specific details can you reveal? Are there ethical obligations that must be considered?*

One piece of legislation that must be considered is HIPAA, the *Health Insurance Portability Accountability Act* (P.L.104-191), passed in 1996.[2] The ethical principle and intent behind HIPAA is of individual autonomy through the protection of medical records and patient privacy. "HIPAA sets a national standard for the protection of certain health information... and assure(s)that individuals' health information is properly protected while allowing the flow of health information needed to provide and promote high quality health care and to protect the public's health and well being."[3] The act details proper patient information management. Violations of the law carry penalties ranging from a $25,000 fine to 10 years in jail and a $250,000 fine, and have also resulted in unpleasant publicity for hospitals and job loss for health care providers.

HIPAA prevents the sharing of identifying patient information without explicit written consent from the patient; this information can include occupation, unique circumstances, age, or other identifying characteristics. It has been argued that if a third party can identify a patient without the name and based solely on the story given, there may be a HIPAA violation. Accordingly, caution must be used in telling advocacy stories where a specific patient might be identified.

RECIPROCITY

Situation/hypothetical. *A new bill that affects emergency medicine is up for deliberation; your representative may cast the deciding vote. You want to advocate for your position on the bill by reminding the candidate of how your emergency medicine organization has supported the candidate in the past. Can you mention past monetary support of the individual candidate or his or her party?*

A novice advocate might be tempted to mention such support; however, lawmakers enacted protection under both federal and state criminal laws. The concept whereby you or your organization have provided past support and now are "due" a vote is called *reciprocity*. The practice also is known as *quid pro quo*, which comes from Latin meaning "something for something." The act is illegal if there is an identifiable exchange between a contribution and a desired action.

A physician can describe his support of the candidates' position and past and present policies, but specific mention of *monetary* contributions should not be made. Legislators and their staff members are well aware of major past contributors, anyhow. Many members of Congress go to the *Republican or Democratic Club* across the street from the legislative offices to hold fundraisers and "dial for dollars" when necessary. You can legally discuss campaign contributions with the member; just be sure not to do it on government property, where such conversations are unethical and technically illegal. Steer away from *quid pro quo*, and you will avoid the ensuing complications.

SOURCES OF ETHICAL GUIDANCE

Where can an emergency physician go for guidance? What resources are available? This section discusses different sources of ethical advocacy.

Emergency Medicine Residents' Association (EMRA)

The Emergency Medicine Residents' Association (EMRA) promotes issues of patient care while representing physician trainees in emergency medicine, who must balance their training and education with employment and workplace issues.[6] An EMRA resolution passed in 2010 promotes advocacy as an integral component of the *Model of the Clinical Practice of Emergency Medicine*.[7] A very similar resolution by the same authors also passed the ACEP Council.

American College of Emergency Physicians (ACEP)

The American College of Emergency Physicians represents approximately 31,000 emergency physicians, residents and medical students. The largest emergency medicine professional organization, ACEP provides perhaps the most detailed ethical guidelines to emergency medicine physicians. The *ACEP Code of Ethics for Emergency Physicians* states that, "The emergency physician owes duties not only to his or her patients, but also to the society in which the physician and patients dwell . . . Emergency physician duties to promote the public health that sometimes transcend duties to individual patients . . . Emergency physicians should be active in legislative, regulatory, institutional, and educational pursuits that promote patient safety and quality emergency care."[8] These are the core principles of emergency physician advocacy.

American Medical Association (AMA)

The American Medical Association seeks to unite physicians nationwide on critical professional and public health issues. AMA policy and ethical guidelines state:

> *"Physicians may participate in individual acts, grassroots activities, or legally permissible collective action to advocate for change. . .physicians must ensure that the health of patients is not jeopardized and that patient care is not compromised. . .Physicians and physicians-in-training should press for needed reforms through the use of informational campaigns, non-disruptive public demonstrations, lobbying and publicity campaigns, and collective negotiation, or other options that do not jeopardize the health of patients or compromise patient care."[9]*

The AMA code also cautions:

> *"In rare circumstances, individual or grassroots actions, such as brief limitations of personal availability, may be appropriate as a means of calling attention to needed changes in patient care. Physicians are cautioned that some actions may put them or their organizations at risk of violating antitrust laws. . ."[10]*

American Bar Association (ABA)

Attorneys who advocate professionally on Capitol Hill are subject to different rules as lobbyists. The rules are useful, in comparison; they demonstrate legal nuances that can serve as a guide. Attorneys acting as lobbyists or engaging the services of a lobbyist are subject to the *Rules of Professional Conduct* that apply to all lawyers. Individual state bar associations' ethical guidelines have "issues opinions" that delineate the ethical guidelines and rules to be followed in advocacy and lobbying. For the physician advocate, knowledgeable attorneys can be a great resource regarding specific ethical concerns requiring further discussion.

NURSING ASSOCIATIONS

American Nurses Association (ANA)

Nurses have been behind some of the most important changes in the U.S. health care system and remain powerful allies in improving medical care for all. *The American Nurses Association* is a professional organization representing 3.1 million registered nurses who advocate for a variety of important issues. The ANA created ethical guidelines similar to those of the American Medical

Association, which state, "Nurses should advance their profession by contributing in some way to the leadership, activities, and the viability of their professional organizations . . . Nurses can also advance the profession through participation in civic activities related to health care or through local, state, national, or international initiatives."[11] Furthermore, nursing educators can promote advocacy: "Nurse educators have a specific responsibility to enhance students' commitment to professional and civic values."[12]

Emergency Nurses Association (ENA)

The Emergency Nurses Association has nearly 40,000 members and continues to grow; its members represent more than 35 countries around the world. ENA seeks to "advocate for patient safety and excellence in emergency nursing practice." The association's code of ethics states the following:[13]

- The emergency nurse acts with compassion and respect for human dignity and the uniqueness of the individual.
- The emergency nurse maintains competence within, and accountability for, emergency nursing practice.
- The emergency nurse acts to protect the individual when health care and safety are threatened by incompetent, unethical or illegal practice.
- The emergency nurse exercises sound judgment in responsibility, delegating, and seeking consultation.
- The emergency nurse respects the individual's right to privacy and confidentiality.
- The emergency nurse works to improve public health and secure access to health care for all.

RUNNING FOR OFFICE

Situation/hypothetical: *You have had a great career as an emergency medicine practitioner, but now want to make more of an impact; you are interested in politics and are considering becoming a representative. What ethical considerations should be made? What conflicts exist, and how can you stay out of trouble?*

Being cognizant of the law is critical to staying out of trouble. For novice politicians with party affiliations, guidance can come from the party. The objective in politics is re-election, whether at the local, state or federal level. Physicians-turned-representatives have many obligations – to the constituency, to society, and to the party. They also have important obligations to their profession; there are codes, charters and rules to which they must adhere. When running for office, candidates may be required to file financing forms and disclose financial interests in election or ethics reports. Financial reporting laws differ from state to state and require detailed investigation prior to embarking on the campaign trail.[14] One must take care in balancing the ramifications of all previous associations and affiliations when running for political appointment.

CONCLUSION

Being politically effective in your advocacy efforts requires skill and attention to ethical principles; such knowledge is fundamental. The examples above illustrate the balance needed between promoting one's specialty and patient protection. Various guidelines have been created by a variety of medical organizations; ethical principles, in combination with a solid legal framework, encourage and protect medical advocacy. A balance of all interests and knowledge of these principles is necessary to becoming an effective advocate of both patients and emergency medicine. Your voice, combined with action, creates change! ✷

Chapter 29

EMERGING MEDICAL TECHNOLOGIES
A Pathway to Improving Quality of Care and Patient Outcomes

Zachary Ginsberg, MD, MPP

> *In the past half-century, all of the following have been in vogue at one time or another: redesigning professional education; improving peer review of physician practice; reengineering systems of care; increasing competition among provider organizations; publicly reporting data on quality; rewarding good performance; punishing bad performance; applying continuous quality improvement or total quality management tools; and measuring and improving the culture of health care organizations to facilitate the adoption of safer systems of care.[1]*

E mergency departments are high-risk environments in which reliable and safe practices are *essential*. In an era of continuous, value-added quality solutions for improving patient care and safety, we must first articulate our goals and vision. Many organizations receive regular reports on potentially unsafe conditions, poorly functioning safety procedures, or simple changes in the environment that may potentially lead to failures of safety systems. It is imperative that patients receive evidence-based, equitable, timely care in a system designed to deliver it. With between 23-44% of health care deemed wasteful, harmful, or inappropriate, medicine has much room for improvement.[2,3]

In the era of the Affordable Care Act, which requires meaningful use of electronic health records, it is important to identify how technology can add value to the clinical setting. This is an exciting time, during which the novel application of existing technologies can result in a streamlined care delivery system; patient results are "pushed" to the clinician and outcomes not only are tracked, but are rendered increasingly predictable with the improvement of statistical analysis.

Innovations and technologies that already exist in other sectors have natural applications to the clinical environment of the emergency department. Many interventions that advance throughput and shorten patient care times risk undermining the quality of care delivered, as health providers rush through each step to improve the current metrics of door-to-doc or total time in department. Greater speed cannot be the only goal, however; meaningful use must also help focus care to prevent cognitive biases, while streamlining clinical decision-making.[4] Adding value removes waste and passively reinforces safety measures by pushing key information to the provider while simultaneously removing distractions and unnecessary steps. (See Table 1)

Table 1. Common Categories of Waste in Health Care

Overproduction	Any health care service that does not add value to the patient
Inventories	Overstocking, inability to find an item, expired products, etc.
Over-processing	Repeated bed moves, redundancies, etc.
Motion of employees	Searching for patients, returning to computers, etc.
Transport of patients	Long transport times or distances
Waiting	Additional waiting once results have been posted, etc.
Error correction	Time lost correcting the error, rather than preventing it in the first place

The adoption of a given program must be matched by its ability to streamline the care required by all emergency physicians to improve patient safety and the quality of care delivered. Reinforcing *passive monitoring* with technology can help prevent cognitive biases and augment clinical decision-making. For example, a recent study on the early identification of sepsis found that the use of technology resulted in more consistent ordering of blood cultures and lactates, but did *not* expedite the diagnosis of patients going in to septic shock.[5] While there were no changes in care times, the findings illustrate that the use of an *electronic medical record* (EMR) can increase the application of evidence-based practices for critical ED patients.

Current EMRs track what *already* has happened to a patient; alternatively, a prospective evidence-based standardized care pathway linked to an EMR could help prompt clinicians regarding their next steps in management.[6] Such passive pathways can increase both efficiency and patient safety. Existing *push technology* to alert clinicians about abnormal labs or high-priority imaging may streamline care. Patients experience expedited throughputs when a system is designed to move them along through their hospital courses.[7]

EMR IN THE EMERGENCY DEPARTMENT

An electronic medical record that archives patient data for return visits in a primary care setting serves a very different purpose than an EMR of a decompensated patient presenting to the ED. It is essential to direct attention toward an ED user interface when designing an EMR. In the fast-paced ED setting, focus quickly toggles between activities; in an ideal EMR, push technology will help the physician triage the many pieces of data and decisions that an emergency physician must handle every day.

Imagine two simultaneous cases for which selective health IT exists and has been implemented. In the first, a 28-year-old male is brought to the ED by EMS after a motor vehicle collision; and in the second, a 62-year-old female presents with acute onset slurred speech and right-sided numbness. The 28-year-old male has diminished breath sounds on the right, and the 62-year-old woman has obvious focal neurological deficits that began within the last hour.

The status of the patients is known even before they approach because the resuscitation bay monitor has the capacity to stream pre-hospital EMS vital signs. Handheld photographs of the collision are provided by EMS on arrival to help reconstruct the vectors of the accident and gauge the severity of impact.

The meaningful use of electronic medical records requires a mindfulness and attention to detail at all levels of health care delivery – from hospital leadership to the clinician at the bedside – to create a culture of safety capable of making robust improvements to patient care through the adoption of novel technologies.

First, both patients are examined and bedside registration occurs. While ABCs are stabilized in the trauma patient, the ED physician activates both the stroke and trauma teams by pushing an alert button on a handheld computerized physician order entry (CPOE) device. The stroke patient is sent quickly to the CT scan; by selecting a priority level, the physician moves the scan to the top of the radiologist's viewing list and will receive an alert once the scan is complete. Prioritization of imaging studies, from the critical to the mundane, seems logical, useful and inevitable as emergency medicine physicians continue to improve the coordination and deployment of highly demanded resources.[8]

While overseeing the trauma, the emergency physician places a streaming video of the stroke patient on a handheld device. *Remote telemetry monitoring* – from either an online medical control or hospital-based system, such as "tele-ICU" (now being piloted at the Steward's Hospitals in Boston, MA)[9] – allows physicians to transmit images and vital signs from a camera at the foot of the bed.[10] Simultaneous monitoring has the unique capability of improving oversight and safety with back-up support from tele-physician physicians, who can suggest medications or catch concerning trends in vital signs. The shift from *static* to *mobile* workstations untethers the emergency physician from the desktop computer space, and reduces the total time spent traveling between locations.

ABCs are performed on the trauma patient showing diminished breath sounds. The pre-setup equipment tray is in place on a mobile cart prior to the patient's arrival, with enough space to set up a sterile field. X-rays have been taken by imaging equipment that drops down from the ceiling. The patient is cleared for CT and wheeled to the scanner; oxygen and telemetry monitoring already is built into the hospital bed.

On the way to the scanner, a push notification on the handheld CPOE alerts the emergency physician that a neurologist is at the bedside and the patient's head CT is complete. As the physician walks into the patient's room, the video monitor switches to display vital signs, while the camera images stream from the trauma patient in the CT scanner. The CT images can be scrolled through on the handheld; the status of the "read" allows the physician to call the radiologist, listen to the dictation, or see the official read. Simultaneously, the emergency physician can order IV tPA through a wireless network that sends the order to the pharmacy and automated medication dispensing system (or Pyxis).

Many patient safety interventions have focused on patient equipment and advances in the method of dispensing medications. If CPOE occurs from a handheld device, all medications are available immediately after a nurse enters the patient name into the automated medication dispensing system. The medications have been crosschecked by the computer and adjusted by the pharmacy to avoid interactions and dosing errors; lights indicate the location of each medication.

Finally, in an effort for continuous quality improvement, recording the care could enrich the debriefing process and enable the health care team to identify opportunities for better coordination, communication and care delivery. Patient outcomes can be assessed, and outcomes that deviate from the norm can be identified more quickly. Every step of this process is charted more easily and time-stamped by bedside CPOE. Errors and complications are identified the moment they occur, and real-time response becomes possible; subsequent root cause analysis also becomes easier, since each step of the process is recorded.

THE ROLE OF EMR IN QUALITY IMPROVEMENT

This scenario highlights the ability of an EMR to record what has is happening to a patient in real-time. Perhaps the greatest potential benefit of EMR, however, is the ability to electronically record a streaming dataset of patient information, acuity and pathology.[11] Statistical models such as *statistical process control* (SPC) and *Bayesian analysis* would allow for predictive modeling of patient demand, in proportion to current hospital capacity, to facilitate the earlier identification of surge events. This improvement in situational awareness could allow emergency physicians to identify problems even before they occur, so preventive measures could be taken.[12] We are far from being able to predict what a given shift will be like prior to heading into work; this may be a possible in the future, however, as we delve into the richness of emergency medical records and the integrated prospective design they offer.

Particularly useful in EMRs are dashboards utilized by administrators to focus on relevant metrics, rather than the indirect measurement of number of patients in the waiting room. Utilizing statistical process control and trend charts can all help to identify when the emergency department is operating in surge conditions long before boarding and crowding grow to dangerous levels, allowing activation of surge contingency plans earlier and limiting the problem's full impact.

The power of these tools lies in their systematic approach, which involves the following: *reliably measuring the magnitude of a problem; identifying the root causes of the problem and measuring the importance of each cause; finding solutions for the most important causes; proving the effectiveness of those solutions; and deploying programs to ensure sustained improvements over time.*[1] Real-time trending through EMRs and smoothing the coordination among and between services can create a culture of collaboration. Specifically, any sentinel event will be caught sooner and addressed more quickly by a constantly updated administration committed to patient safety and the delivery of quality care.

At every stage of quality improvement, we must look for opportunities to promote value and reduce waste and harm.[1,4] The goal of electronic health records is to improve patient safety and ease the sharing of information;[2] EMRs also may help improve patient flow without compromising safety – the holy grail of emergency medicine. Technology in health care – and in other sectors, selectively applied to the ED – may bring about meaningful change.

As charting and hospital processes become increasingly real-time, opportunities arise for immediate bed assignments and anticipation of admission, based on validated criteria (such as complexity of the work-up as it occurs, or combinations of medications that typically lead to admissions).[13,14] In our patient examples, the placement of a chest tube and the order for IV tPA could have reduced wait time and prompted the hospital to identify a likely admission and begin preparing an appropriate bed.

Policymakers have made considerable financial and legal investments to implement the integrated electronic medical records and care pathways described above. As part of the 2009 stimulus package, the federal government spent $30 billion, primarily through physician incentives, to accelerate the adoption of EMRs; measures to improve patient safety are required for an EMR to meet the criteria required for meaningful use.[2,15,16] The use of health information technology to develop an emergency department-specific electronic health record has the potential to improve care and patient outcomes significantly. Better recording of care delivery can help providers safely multitask and can improve the review of adverse events.

CONCLUSION

The ability of health information technology to prospectively predict the needs of patients and hospitals, including outcomes and recommended management algorithms, has the greatest potential to improve care in *real time*. Simply translating the same practices one employed on paper to an electronic format does not improve the delivery of care; it only replicates already existing health care delivery problems and misses the opportunity to *predict*, rather than merely *record*, patient experiences. The meaningful use of electronic medical records requires a mindfulness and attention to detail at all levels of health care delivery – from hospital leadership to the clinician at the bedside – to create a culture of safety capable of making robust improvements to patient care.[14] ✱

AFTERWORD

By reading this handbook, you have expanded your understanding of the issues that currently face emergency physicians and patients beyond the clinical realm. Armed with that knowledge, you can be an effective voice for your patients on the local, state, and national levels. Solutions to the challenges we face are not simple, but awareness of these issues is the first step in being able to advocate for improvement.

The future of medicine and the practice of emergency medicine fundamentally will change within our lifetimes. Each of us should be *involved*, working collaboratively to shape this future for emergency physicians and patients. Learn how to get involved, and use the chapters in this handbook as a resource when an issue inspires you. EMRA will keep you informed and seek your involvement as issues come to the forefront. Join us as we rise to meet these challenges, and help populate the next generation of leaders in our specialty. ✱

Nathan R. Schlicher, MD, JD, FACEP and Alison Haddock, MD

CHAPTER REFERENCES

Chapter 2 References

1. Rabin E et al., Solutions to Emergency Department 'Boarding ' and Crowding Are Underused and May Need to Be Legislated. *Health Affairs* 2012:31(8): 1757-66 (quoting U.S. Institute of Medicine, Hospital-based Emergency Care: At the Breaking Point. National Academies Press, 2006.

2. The latest number is 136.1 million in 2009, per the CDC, available at http://www.cdc.gov/nchs/fastats/ervisits.htm referencing National Hospital Ambulatory Medical Care Survey: 2009 Emergency Department Summary Tables, Table 1, available at http://www.cdc.gov/nchs/data/ahcd/nhamcs_emergency/2009_ed_web_tables.pdf. This is up from 116.8 million in 2007. Tang N et al., Trans and Characteristics of U.S. Emergency Department Visits, 1997-2007. *JAMA* 2010:304(6): 664-70.

3. However, in the long term healthcare reform under the Affordable Care Act may lead to decreased emergency room visits. *See, e.g.*, Long SK et al., Massachusetts Health Reforms: Uninsurance Remains Low, Self- Reported Health Status Improves As State Prepares to Tackle Costs. *Health Affairs* 2012:31(2): 1-8 (showing that emergency department visits for adults ages 19-64 dropped between Fall 2006-Fall 2010 for the first time in the fall of 2010, a finding corroborated by analysis of the state's administrative data.).

4. Increasing inpatient capacity does not necessarily mean more beds; it could be achieved through things such as improving bed turnover or changing the availability of ancillary services. See, e.g., Rabin *supra* note 1.

5. Derlet RW & Richards JR. Overcrowding in the Nation's Emergency Departments: Complex Causes and Disturbing Effects. *Ann Emerg Med.* 2000:35(1): 63-8.

6. Gibbs N. Do you want to die? The crisis in emergency care is taking its toll on doctors, nurses, and patients. *Time.* May 28, 1990: 58-65.

7. Institute of Medicine. Hospital-Based Emergency Care: At the Breaking Point. Executive Summary. The National Academies Press, 2007.

8. Asplin BR et al., A Conceptual Model of Emergency Department Crowding. *Ann Emerg Med* 2003:42(2):173-80.

9. Niska R, Bhuiya F, & Xu J. National Hospital Ambulatory Medical Care Survey: 2007 Emergency Department Summary. National Health Statistics Reports, 2010 August 6; (26): 1-32.

10. *See* National Hospital Ambulatory Medical Care Survey, *supra* note 2.

11. Government Accountability Office. Emergency Departments: Unevenly Affected by Growth and Change in Patient Use. Washington: US General Accounting Office; 1993 January 24.

12. Sommers A, Boukus E, & Carrier E. Dispelling Myths About Emergency Department Use: Majority of Medicaid Visits Are for Urgent or More Serious Symptoms. Center for Studying Health Systems Change, HSC Research Brief No. 23; 2012.

13. Cunningham, P. Nonurgent Use of Hospital Emergency Departments. Statement Before the U.S. Senate Health, Education, Labor and Pensions Committee Subcommittee on Primary Health and Aging at 6, May, 2011 (stating that only 8% of ED visits in 2008 could be classified as nonurgent based on triage symptoms).

14. Roberts DC, McKay MP & Shaffer A. Increasing Rates of Emergency Department Visits for Elderly Patients in the United States, 1993 to 2003. *Ann Emerg Med.* 2008:51(6): 769-74.

15. Pitts SR et al., Where Americans Get Acute Care: Increasingly, It's not at Their Doctor's Office. *Health Affairs* 2010:29(9): 1620-29 (finding that 28% of acute care visits occur in the ED).

16. Berry, E. Emergency Department Volume Rises as Office Visits Fall. American Medical News, Jan 16, 2012 *available at* www.amednews.com/article/20120116/business/301169965/6/

17. Schull MJ, Kiss A & Szalai JP. The Effect of Low-Complexity Patients on Emergency Department Waiting Times. *Ann Emerg Med* 2007:49(3): 257-64.

18. *See, e.g.*, Courtemanche CJ & Zapata D. Does Universal Coverage Improve Health? The Massachusetts Experience, NEBR Working Paper 17893 (March 2012), available at http://www.nber.org/papers/w17893. *See also* Finklestein A et al., The Oregon Health Insurance Experiment: Evidence from the First Year, NBER Working Paper 17190 (2011), available at http://www.nber.org/papers/w17190.pdf; Baiker K & Finklestein A, The Effects of Medicaid Coverage – Learning from the Oregon Experiment, *N Eng J Med* 2012:365(8): 683-85.

19. American Hospital Association, Chartbook: Trends Affecting Hospital and Health Systems. Table 3.3: Emergency Department Visits, Emergency Department Visits per 1000, and Number of Emergency Departments, 1999-2010, *available at* www.aha.org/research/reports/tw/chartbook/2012/table3-3.pdf. *See also* Tang N *supra* note 2 (discussing the decrease in the number of Emergency Departments).

20. American Hospital Association, American Hospital Association Statistics, available at www.healthforum.com & American Hospital Association. Fast Facts on US Hospitals, *available at available a*t: http://www.aha.org/research/rc/stat-studies/fast-facts.shtml.

21. American Hospital Association, Annual Survey of Hospitals, Table 116, available at http://www.cdc.gov/nchs/data/hus/2011/116.pdf.

22. McCaig LF et al. Estimates of Emergency Department Capacity: United States, 2007, National Center for Health Statistics, *available at* http://www.cdc.gov/nchs/data/hestat/ed_capacity/ed_capacity.htm.

23. Government Accountability Office. Hospital Emergency Departments: Crowded Conditions Vary among Hospitals and Communities. Washington: US General Accounting Office; 2003. The definition of timely varies. Less than 2 hours from admission order is one definition, which is what the Government Accountability Office used in its report. See also Welch S et al. Emergency Department Performance Measures and Benchmarking Summit. *Acad Emerg Med* 2006:13(10): 1074-80.

24. Litvak E et al. Emergency Department Diversion: Causes and Solutions. *Acad Emerg Med.* 2001:8(10):1108-10.

25. Moskop JC et al. Emergency Department Crowding, Part 1 – Concept, Causes, and Moral Consequences. *Ann Emerg Med.* 2009:53(5): 605-11.

26. Richardson DB. The Access Block Effect: Relationship between Delay to Reaching an Inpatient Bed and Inpatient Length of Stay. *Med J Aust* 2002:177(9): 492-5.

27. Forster AJ et al. The Effect of Hospital Occupancy on Emergency Department Length of Stay and Patient Disposition. *Acad Emerg Med.* 2003:10(2): 127-33.

28. *See* Rabin *supra* note 1.

29. *See* GAO *supra* note 24.

30. *See* IOM *supra* note 1.

31. *See* Forster *supra* note 28.

32. Falvo T et al. The Opportunity Loss of Boarding Admitted Patients in the Emergency Department. *Acad Emerg Med* 2007:14(4):332-7.

33. American College of Emergency Physicians Task Force on Boarding. Emergency Department Crowding: High Impact Solutions. 2008, available at www.acep.org/workarea/DownloadAsset.aspx?id=50026.

34. Bernstein SL et al. The Effect of Emergency Department Crowding on Clinically Oriented Outcomes, *Acad Emerg Med* 2009:16(1): 1-10.
35. CDC. QuickStats: Percentage of Emergency Department Visits with Waiting Time for a Physician of > 1 Hour, by Race/Ethnicity and Triage Level – United States, 2003-2004. *MMWR Weekly.* 2006:55(16): 463.
36. Wilson J & Wein D. Boarding Times and Patient Safety: a Generalizable Quantitative Model. ACEP 2010 Scientific Assembly; September 28–October 1, 2010; Las Vegas, NV.
37 Richardson DB & Bryant M. Confirmation of Association between Overcrowding and Adverse Events in Patients Who Do Not Wait to be Seen. *Acad Emerg Med.* 2004:11(5): 462.
38. Pines JM & Hollander JE. Association between Cardiovascular Complications and ED crowding. ACEP 2007 Scientific Assembly; October 8-11, 2007; Seattle, WA.
39. Miro O et al. Decreased Health Care Quality Associated with Emergency Department Overcrowding. *Eur J Emerg Med* 1999:6(2): 105-7.
40. Cowan RM & Trzeciak S. Clinical Review: Emergency Department Overcrowding and the Potential Impact on the Critically Ill. *Crit Care.* 2005:9(3): 291-95.
41. Liu SW et al. A Pilot Study Examining Undesired Events Among Emergency Department-Boarded Patients Awaiting Inpatient Beds. *Annals of Emerg Med.* 2009:54(3): 382-85.
42. Krochmal P & Riley TA. Increased Health Care Costs Associated with ED Overcrowding. *Am J Emerg Med.* 1994:12(3): 265-66.
43. *See* Richardson *supra* note 27.
44. Liew D, Liew D & Kennedy MP. Emergency Department Length of Stay Independently Predicts Excess Inpatient Length of Stay. *Med J Aust.* 2003:179(10): 524-26.
45. Singer AJ et al. The Association Between Length of Emergency Department Boarding and Mortality. *Acad Emerg Med.* 2011:18(12): 1324-29.
46. Sprivulis PC et al. The Association Between hospital Overcrowding and Mortality Among Patients Admitted via Western Australian Emergency Departments. *Med J Aust.* 2006:184(5): 208-12.
47. Richardson DB. Increase in Patient Mortality at 10 days Associated with Emergency Department Overcrowding. *Med J Aust.* 2006:184(5): 213-16.
48. Chalfin DB et al. Impact of Delayed Transfer of Critically Ill Patients from the Emergency Department to the Intensive Care Unit. *Crit Care Med.* 2007:35(6):1477-83.
49. *See* Singer *supra* note 46.
50. Burt CW & McCaig LF. Staffing, Capacity, and Ambulance Diversion in Emergency Departments: United States, 2003–04. Advance Data from Vital and Health Statistics, 2006; September 27 (376): 1- 24.
51. *See* ACEP *supra* note 34.
52. *See* Falvo *supra* note 33.
53. Browne BJ & Kuo DC. Patients Admitted through Emergency Department are More Profitable than Patients Admitted Electively. *Ann Emerg Med.* 2004:44(4): s132.
54. Henneman PL et al. Emergency Department Admissions are More Profitable than Non-Emergency Department Admissions. *Ann Emerg Med* 2009:53(2): 249–55.
55. *See* Rabin *supra* note 1.
56. Mitka M. Economics May Play Role in Crowding, Boarding in Emergency Departments. *JAMA* 2008:300(23): 2714-5.
57. McHugh M, Reginstein M & Siegel B. The Profitability of Medicare Admissions Based on Source of Admission. *Acad Emerg Med* 2008:15(10): 900-7.
58. Mountain D. Introduction of a 4-hour Rule in Western Australian Emergency Departments. *Emerg Med Australas* 2010:22(5): 374–8.
59. Weber E et al. Emptying the Corridors of Shame: Organizational Lessons from England's 4-hour Emergency Throughput Target. *Ann Emerg Med.* 2011:57(2): 79–88.

60. Buckley et al. Impact of an Express Admit Unit on Emergency Department Length of Stay. *J Emerg Med* 2010:39(5): 669–73.

61. It should be noted that coverage itself does not equate access or decreased emergency department utilization. However, coverage by itself has been shown to improve health and health outcomes, both subjectively and objectively. *See* Finklestein *supra* note 19; Sommers BD et al. Mortality and Access to are among Adults after State Medicaid Expansions, *N Engl J Med* 2012:367(11): 1025-34; & Courtemanche CJ & Zapata D, Does Universal Coverage Improve Health? The Massachusetts Experience, NEBR Working Paper 17893 (March 2012), available at http://www.nber.org/papers/w17893.

62. Medicaid data from NC and DE show that connecting these traditionally challenging populations with primary care physicians decreased emergency department utilization. *See* Hurley RE et al. Gatekeeping the Emergency Department: Impact of a Medicaid Primary Care Case Management Program, *Health Care Management Rev.* 1989:14(2): 63-71; Gill JM & Diamond JJ, Effect of Primary Care Referral on Emergency Use: Evaluation of a Statewide Medicaid Program, *Del. Med. J.* 1996:68(9): 437-42; & Piehl MD et al. "Narrowing the Gap:" Decreasing Emergency Department Use by Children Enrolled in the Medicaid Program by Improving Access to Primary Care, *Arch Pediatr. Adolesc. Med.* 2000:9(8): 791-5.

63. The literature demonstrates that social and economic factors affect patients' health, health outcomes, and access to healthcare. Addressing these factors can help "optimize" patients for when they do present at the ED, decreasing the need for admission, thus helping with the boarding problem.

64. There are many programs, especially in pediatrics, that address these issues. See, e.g., Zuckerman et al., Why Pediatricians Needs Lawyers to Keep Children Healthy. *Pediatrics* 2004:114(1): 224-8. *See also* Health Leads, https://healthleadsusa.org.

65. Henry J Kaiser Family Foundation. The Uninsured and the Difference Health Insurance Makes. 2010, available at http://www.kff.org/uninsured/1420.cfm.

66 Association of American Medical Colleges. Physician Shortages to Worsen Without Increases in Residency Training. 2010, available at https://www.aamc.org/newsroom/newsreleases/2010/150570/100930.html.

67. Pitts SR et al. Where Americans Get Acute Care: Increasingly It's Not at Their Doctor's Office. *Health Affairs.* 2010:29(9):1620-29.

68. Long SK & Stockley K. Massachusetts Health Reform Survey Policy Brief. Emergency Department Visits in Massachusetts: Who Uses Emergency Care and Why. Robert Wood Johnson Foundation, 2009.

69. Long SK, Stockley K & Dahlen H. Massachusetts Health Reforms: Uninsurance Remains Low, Self-Reported Health Status Improves As State Prepares to Tackle Costs. *Health Affairs* 2012: Webfirst, available at http://content.healthaffairs.org/content/early/2012/01/24/hlthaff.2011.0653.full.html.

70. Miller S. The Effect of Insurance on Emergency Room Visits: An Analysis of the 2006 Massachusetts Health Reform, forthcoming *J. Public Economics,* available at https://netfiles.uiuc.edu/smille36/www/research.html.

71. Cheung D et al. The State of Emergency Medicine Quality Measures. *ACEP News.* November 11, 2011.

Chapter 3 References

1. Conover, Christopher J. *Costs and Benefits of EMTALA.* Center For Health Policy, Duke University. June 2006.
2. P.L. 99-272, 100 Stat. 164 (1986) codified at 42 U.S.C. § 1395dd et seq. (2007).
3. 42 U.S.C. § 1395dd(a). A dedicated emergency department is defined as any facility that is licensed or held out to the public as such, or that provides urgent care to one third of its outpatients during the preceding calendar year. 42 C.F.R. § 489.24(b).
4. Rosenbaum S, Cartwright-Smith L, Hirsh J, Mehler PS. Case Studies At Denver Health: 'Patient Dumping' In The Emergency Department Despite EMTALA, The Law That Banned It. *Health Aff (Millwood).* Aug 2012;31(8):1749-56.
5. The new final EMTALA regulation on EMTALA. 68 Fed. Reg. 53,221-53264 (2003).
6. The new final EMTALA regulation on EMTALA. 68 Fed. Reg. 53,221-53264 (2003).
7. http://www.nytimes.com/2012/08/15/business/hca-giant-hospital-chain-creates-a-windfall-for-private-equity.html?pagewanted=all&_r=0
8. 42 U.S.C. § 1395dd(b)(1) and 42 C.F.R. § 489.24(a)(1)(ii).
9. Bryant v. Adventist, *infra* note 28 at 1166.
10. Emergency Medical Treatment and Active Labor Act, 42 USC 1395dd. http://www.gpo.gov/fdsys/pkg/USCODE-2010-title42/pdf/USCODE-2010-title42-chap7-subchapXVIII-partE-sec1395dd.pdf. Accessed September 14, 2012.
11. 42 C.F.R. § 489.24(b).
12. Naradzay JF, Wood J. *Cobra Laws and EMTALA.* http://emedicine.medscape.com/article/790053-overview.
13. *Moses v. Providence Hospital and Medical Centers, Inc.* 561 F.3d 573 (6th Circuit, 2009).
14. 77 Fed. Reg. 22:5213-5217. Accessible at http://www.gpo.gov/fdsys/pkg/FR-2012-02-02/pdf/2012-2287.pdf
15. Emergency Medical Treatment and Active Labor Act, 42 USC 1395dd. http://www.gpo.gov/fdsys/pkg/USCODE-2010-title42/pdf/USCODE-2010-title42-chap7-subchapXVIII-partE-sec1395dd.pdf. Accessed September 14, 2012.
16. Emergency Medical Treatment and Active Labor Act, 42 USC 1395dd. http://www.gpo.gov/fdsys/pkg/USCODE-2010-title42/pdf/USCODE-2010-title42-chap7-subchapXVIII-partE-sec1395dd.pdf. Accessed September 14, 2012.
17. Emergency Medical Treatment and Active Labor Act, 42 USC 1395dd. http://www.gpo.gov/fdsys/pkg/USCODE-2010-title42/pdf/USCODE-2010-title42-chap7-subchapXVIII-partE-sec1395dd.pdf. Accessed September 14, 2012.
18. Bitterman R. *EMTALA: Emergency Medicine Risk Management.* Irving, TX: American College of Emergency Physicians; 1997: 353-377.
19. Fosmire S. *EMTALA FAQ.* http://emtala.com/faq.htm 71.
20. http://www.acep.org/advocacy/dear-colleague-9-22-2011
21. Niska R, Bhuiya F, Xu J. National Hospital Ambulatory Medical Care Survey: 2009 emergency department summary. Natl Health Stat Report 2010;(26):1–31. 2010.
22. Institute of Medicine, Committee on the Future of Emergency Care in the U.S. Health System. Hospital-based emergency care: at the breaking point. Washington, DC: National Academy of Sciences; 2006.
23. Simonet D. Cost reduction strategies for emergency services: insurance role, practice changes and patients accountability. *Health Care Anal* 2009;17:1–19.
24. Bitterman RA. Explaining the EMTALA paradox. *Ann Emerg Med* 2002;40:470.
25. The Henry J. Kaiser Family Foundation. *The Uninsured: A Primer.* http://kff.org/uninsured/upload/7451-04.pdf
26. *Health Forum, AHA Annual Survey Data, 1980-2009,* accessed at www.aha.org/content/00-10/10uncompensatedcare.pdf

27. Institute of Medicine. *The Future of Emergency Care Report*. Washington, DC: GPO; 2006.
28. American Medical Association and Center for Health Policy Research. *Physician Marketplace Report: The Impact of EMTALA on Physician Practices*. February 2003.
29. Elmendorf D. *Cost Estimate for th Amendment in the Nature of a Substitute for HR 4872*.
30. Buettgens M, et al. *America Under the Affordable Care Act*. Urban Institute, Robert Wood Johnson Foundation. http://www.rwjf.org/files/research/71555.pdf
31. Patient Protection and Affordable Care Act (PPACA), § 3133 as amended by PPACA, § 10316 and as further amended by § 1104 of the Health Care and Education Reconciliation Act (HCERA), P.L. No. 111-152 (Mar. 30, 2010).
32. HR. 157 (ih). Health Care Safety Net Enhancement Act of 2011. http://www.gpo.gov/fdsys/pkg/BILLS-112hr157ih/pdf/BILLS-112hr157ih.pdf.

Chapter 4 References

1. National Center for Health Statistics. *National Hospital Ambulatory Medical Care Survey: 2009 Emergency Department Summary Tables*. Hyattsville, MD: Center for Disease Control and Prevention.
2. Agency for Healthcare Research and Quality. *Medical Expenditure Panel Survey*. Rockville, MD: Department of Health and Human Services; 2008.
3. Government Accountability Office. *Emergency Departments Unevenly Affected by Growth and Change in Patient Use*. HRD-93-4. January 1993.
4. Niska R, Bhuiya F, and Xu J. (National Center for Health Statistics). *National Hospital Ambulatory Medical Care Survey: 2007 Emergency Department Summary*. Hyattsville, MD: Center for Disease Control and Prevention; 2010.
5. Garcia TC, Bernstein AB, Bush MA. (National Center for Health Statistics). *Emergency department visitors and visits: Who used the emergency room in 2007?* Hyattsville, MD: Center for Disease Control and Prevention; 2010.
6. Zink B. *Anyone, Anything, Anytime: A History of Emergency Medicine*. Mosby, 2006.
7. Hsia RY et al. Do mandates requiring insurers to pay for emergency care influence the use of the emergency department? *Health Affairs*. 2006;25(4): 1086-1094.
8. Hall MA. The impact and enforcement of prudent layperson laws. *Ann Emerg Med*. 2004:43(5): 558-566.
9. P.L. 105-33: To provide for reconciliation pursuant to subsections (b)(1) and (c) of section 015 of the concurrent resolution on the budget for fiscal year 1998 (8/5/97; enacted HR 2015).
10. P.L 111-148: Entitled the Patient Protection and Affordable Care Act (3/23/10; enacted HR 3590).
11. Celeste, J. The Method Behind the Madness: Examining the Tool that States are Misusing to Limit ED Visits. *EM Resident*. 2012;39(2): 8-9.
12. Billings J et al. Emergency Room Use: The New York Story. The Commonwealth Fund, November 2000.

Chapter 5 References

1. Emergency Medical Treatment and Active Labor Act, established under the Consolidated Omnibus Budget Reconciliation Act of 1985. *Pub L* No. 99-272, 42USC 1395dd (1986).
2. Weiner, R. "Romney: Uninsured have emergency rooms." *Washington Post*, Sept 24, 2012. Access online on October 18, 2012 at: http://www.washingtonpost.com/blogs/election-2012/wp/2012/09/24/romney-calls-emergency-room-a-health-care-option-for-uninsured
3. Foster R. Memorandum on estimated financial effects of the 'Patient Protection and Affordable Care Act.' Centers for Medicare and Medicaid Services, Office of the Actuary. April 22, 2010.
4. Niska R, Bhuiya F, Xu J. National Hospital Ambulatory Medical Care Survey: 2007 Emergency Department Summary. National Health Statistics Reports. 2012; 26: 1-31.
5. ACEP News Release: Emergency Visits Are Increasing, New Poll Finds; Many Patients Referred by Primary Care Doctors. April 28, 2011.
6. Massachusetts Division of Healthcare Policy and Financing. Hospital inpatient and emergency department utilization trends fiscal years 2004-2008. [Online]. Available at http://www.mass.gov. 2010; [Accessed August, 2010].
7. Hing E, Bhuiya F. NCHS Data Brief: Wait Time for Treatment in Hospital Emergency Departments: 2009. Number 102, August 2012.
8. Hsia R, Kellermann A, Shen Y. Factors associated with closures of emergency departments in the United States. *JAMA*. 2011;305(19):1978-1985. doi:10.1001/jama.2011.620.
9. Sun BC, et al. Effects of hospital closures and hospital characteristics on emergency department ambulance diversion, Los Angeles County, 1998 to 2004. *Annals of Emergency Medicine*. 2007; 47(4):309-315.
10. Huang J, Silbert J, Regenstein M. America's Public Hospitals and Health Systems, 2003: Results of the Annual NAPH Hospital Characteristics Survey. 2005; Washington, DC: National Association of Public Hospitals and Health Systems.
11. Focus on Health Reform: Summary of New Health Reform Law. Kaiser Family Foundation, April 15, 2011.
12. National Hospital Ambulatory Medical Care Survey: 2009 Emergency Department Summary Tables. CDC. Accessed online October 18, 2012 at: http://www.cdc.gov/nchs/data/ahcd/nhamcs_emergency/2009_ed_web_tables.pdf
13. Sanders AB. Older persons in the emergency medical care system. *J Am Geriatr Soc* 2001;49:1390–1392.
14. Wofford JL, Schwartz E, Timerding BL, et al. Emergency department utilization by the elderly: analysis of the National Hospital Ambulatory Medical Care Survey. *Acad Emerg Med*. 1996;3:694-699.
15. McNamara RM , Rousseau E , Sanders AB. Geriatric emergency medicine: a survey of practicing emergency physicians. *Annals of Emerg Med*. 1992;21:796–801.
16. Samaras N, Chevalley T, Samaras D, Gold G. Older patients in the emergency department: a review. *Ann Emerg Med*. 2010;56:261-269.
17. Grossmann FF, Zumbrunn T, Frauchiger A, Delport K, Bingisser R, Nickel CH. At risk of undertriage? Testing the performance and accuracy of the emergency severity index in older emergency department patients. *Ann Emerg Med*. 2012; 60(3):317-25.e3. doi: 10.1016/j.annemergmed.2011.12.013. Epub 2012 Mar 7.
18. Hwang U, Morrison RS. The geriatric emergency department. *J Am Geriatr Soc*. 2007 Nov;55(11):1873-6.
19. Berger, E. Geriatric emergency department targets aging population: Specialized unit for the aged. *Annals of Emergency Medicine*. 2009; 54 (1):23A-25A.
20. Ginde AA, Sullivan AF, Camargo CA Jr. National study of the emergency physician workforce, 2008. *Ann Emerg Med*. 2009; Sep;54(3):349-59.

21. Camargo CA Jr, Ginde AA, Singer AH, Espinola JA, Sullivan AF, Pearson JF, Singer AJ. Assessment of emergency physician workforce needs in the United States, 2005. *Acad Emerg Med.* 2008; Dec;15(12):1317-20.
22. NHT (Nurses for a Healthier Tomorrow). Emergency Nurse. [Online]. Available: http://www.nursesource.org/emergency.html. 2006. Accessed August, 2010.
23. Burerhaus, P, Staider, D, Auerback, D. The future of the nursing workforce in the United States: Data, trends, and implications. 2008; Boston, MA: Jones & Bartlett
24. American College of Emergency Physicians (ACEP). On-call specialist coverage in U.S. emergency departments: ACEP survey of emergency department directors. [Online]. Available at www.acep.org. 2006. Accessed August, 2010.
25. Green L, Melnick GA, Nawathe A. On-Call Physicians at California Emergency Departments: Problems and Potential Solutions. 2005; Oakland, CA: California Healthcare Foundation.
26. O'Malley AS, Gerland AM, Pham HH, Berenson RA. Rising Pressure: Hospital Emergency Departments: Barometers of the Health Care System. 2005; Washington, DC: The Center for Studying Health System Change.
27. Middleton KR, Burt CW. Availability of Pediatric Services and Equipment in Emergency Departments: United States, 2002-03. 2006; Hyattsville, MD: National Center for Health Statistics.
28. Moorhead JC, Gallery ME, Hirshkorn C, Barnaby DP, Barsan WG, Conrad LC, Dalsey WC, Fried M, Herman SH, Hogan P, Mannle TE, Packard DC, Perina DG, Pollack CV Jr, Rapp MT, Rorrie CC Jr, Schafermeyer RW. A study of the workforce in emergency medicine: 1999. *Annals of Emergency Medicine.* 2002; 40(1):3–15.
29. Sklar D, Spencer D, Alcock J, Cameron S, Saiz M. Demographic analysis and needs assessment of rural emergency departments in New Mexico (DANARED–NM*). Annals of Emergency Medicine.* 2002; 39(4):456–457.
30. Svenson JE, Spurlock C, Nypaver M. Factors associated with the higher traumatic death rate among rural children. *Annals of Emergency Medicine.* 1996; 27(5):625–632.
31. Rogers FB, Osler TM, Shackford SR, Morrow PL, Sartorelli KH, Camp L, Healey MA, Martin F. A population-based study of geriatric trauma in a rural state. *Journal of Trauma-Injury Infection & Critical Care.* 2001. 50(4):604–609.
32. Branas CC, et al. Access to trauma centers in the United States. *JAMA.* 2005; 293(21):2626-33.

Chapter 6 References

1. DeNavas-Walt C, Proctor BD, and Smith JC. Income, Poverty, and Health Insurance Coverage in the United States: 2010. In: Bureau USC, ed. Washington, DC: U.S. Government Printing Office; 2011:60-239.
2. The Kaiser Family Foundation KFF. Cumulative Increases in Health Insurance Premiums, Workers' Contributions to Premiums, Inflation, and Workers' Earnings, 1999-2012. 9/11/2012. Available at: http://facts.kff.org/chart.aspx?ch=2834. Accessed 1/20/2013.
3. Reinhardt UE. Is Employer-Based Health Insurance Worth Saving? *The New York Times.* New York; 2009.
4. National Health Expenditures 2010 Highlights. Department of Health and Human Services, Centers for Medicare & Medicaid Services; 2011.
5. The Board of Trustees FHIaFSM, Funds IT. 2012 Annual Report In: Treasury USDot, ed. Washington, D.C.: United States Government Printing Office; 2012.
6. Christopher J. Truffer JDK, Christian J. Wolfe, Kathryn E. Rennie, Jessica F. Shuff. 2012 Actuarial Report on the Financial Outlook for Medicaid. In: Office of the Actuary CfMMS, Department of Health and Human Services, ed.: US Government Printing Office; 2012.

7. Office CB. Estimates for the Insurance Coverage Provisions of the Affordable Care Act Updated for the Recent Supreme Court Decision. Washington, DC: U.S. Government Printing Office; 2012.

8. Barbara S. Klees CJW, and Catherine A. Curtis. Brief Summaries of Medicare & Medicaid. In: Office of the Actuary CfMMS, Department of Health and Human Services, ed. Washington, DC; 2012.

9. DeNavas-Walt C, Proctor BD, and Smith JC. Income, Poverty, and Health Insurance Coverage in the United States: 2011. In: Bureau USC, ed. Washington, DC: U.S. Government Printing Office; 2012.

10. Department of Veterans Affairs. FY 2013 President's Budget. U.S. Government Printing Office; 2012.

11. Roubideaux Y. Fiscal Year 2013 Budget Justification. In: Indian Health Service DoHaHS, ed.: US Government Printing Office; 2012.

12. Sommers BD. Number of Young Adults Gaining Insurance Due to the Affordable Care Act Now Tops 3 Million. In: Evaluation OotASfPa, ed.: U.S. Government Printing Office; 2012.

13. Estimates for the Insurance Coverage Provisions of the Affordable Care Act Updated for the Recent Supreme Court Decision. Washington, DC: U.S. Government Printing Office; 2012.

14. Kaiser Commission on Medicaid and the Uninsured. *The Uninsured: A Primer. Key facts about Americans without health insurance.* The Kaiser Family Foundation; 2012.

15. National Center for Health Statistics (U.S.). National Hospital Ambulatory Medical Care Survey: 2009 Emergency Department Summary Tables. *DHHS publication.* Hyattsville, Md.: U.S. Dept. of Health and Human Services, Public Health Service, Centers for Disease Control and Prevention; 2009:v.

16. Tang N, Stein J, Hsia RY, et al. Trends and characteristics of U.S. emergency department visits, 1997-2007. *JAMA.* Aug 11 2010;304(6):664-670.

17. Newton MF, Keirns CC, Cunningham R, et al. Uninsured adults presenting to US emergency departments: assumptions vs data. *JAMA.* Oct 22 2008;300(16):1914-1924.

18. Asplin BR, Rhodes KV, Levy H, et al. Insurance status and access to urgent ambulatory care follow-up appointments. *JAMA.* Sep 14 2005;294(10):1248-1254.

19. Access of Medicaid recipients to outpatient care. *N Engl J Med.* May 19 1994;330(20): 1426-1430.

20. Mortensen K, Song PH. Minding the gap: a decomposition of emergency department use by Medicaid enrollees and the uninsured. *Med Care.* Oct 2008;46(10):1099-1107.

21. Sommers AS, Boukus ER, Carrier E. Dispelling myths about emergency department use: majority of Medicaid visits are for urgent or more serious symptoms. *Res Brief.* Jul 2012(23):1-10, 11-13.

21a. Chen C, Scheffler G, Chandra A. Massachusetts' Health Care Reform and Emergency Department Utilization. *N Engl J Med.* Sep 2011; 365:e25.

22. LaCalle E, Rabin E. Frequent users of emergency departments: the myths, the data, and the policy implications. *Ann Emerg Med.* Jul 2010;56(1):42-48.

23. Doupe MB, Palatnick W, Day S, et al. Frequent users of emergency departments: developing standard definitions and defining prominent risk factors. *Ann Emerg Med.* Jul 2012;60(1):24-32.

24. Smulowitz PB, Lipton R, Wharam JF, et al. Emergency department utilization after the implementation of Massachusetts health reform. *Ann Emerg Med.* Sep 2011;58(3):225-234 e221.

25. Authority CHIC. Commonwealth Care Health Benefits and Copayments. Boston, MA; 2012.

Chapter 7 References

1. Henry J. Kaiser Family Foundation (KFF). Fact Sheet. Trends in Health Care Costs and Spending (2009). March 2009.
2. LaVeist, Thomas A., Darrell J. Gaskin, and Patrick Richard. The Economic Burden of Health Inequalities in the United States (2009). The Joint Center for Political and Economic Studies, Johns Hopkins University and the University of Maryland. September 2009.
3. Henry J. Kaiser Family Foundation (KFF). Facts on Health Reform. Health Reform and Communities of Color: Implications for racial and ethnic health disparities (2010). September 2010.
4. World Health Organization (WHO), Commission on Social Determinants of Health. "Closing the gap in a generation: Health equity through action on the social determinants of health." Final Report. Executive Summary. 2008.
5. Hebert, Paul L., Sisk, Jane E., Howell Elizabeth A (2008). When Does A Difference Become A Disparity? Conceptualizing Racial And Ethnic Disparities In Health. Health Affairs, 27(2):374-382.
6. Whitehead, Margaret. The concepts and principles of equity and health. Health Promotion International (1991) 6(3): 217-228. (As prepared for the Programme on Health Policies and Planning of the WHO Regional Office for Europe).
7. Institute of Medicine (IOM). Unequal treatment: Confronting racial and ethnic disparities in health. Washington: National Academies Press; 2003.
8. 42 U.S.C. United States Code, 2003 Edition. Title 42. The Public Health and Welfare. Chapter 6A. Public Health Service. Subchapter VII. Agency for Healthcare Research and Quality. Part A – Establishment and General Duties. Sec. 299a-1 – Research on health disparities.
9. 42 U.S.C. United States Code, 2003 Edition. Title 42. The Public Health and Welfare. Chapter 6A. Public Health Service. Subchapter VII. Agency for Healthcare Research and Quality. Part B – Health Care Improvement Research. Sec. 299b-2 – Information on quality and cost of care.
10. Agency for Healthcare Research and Quality (AHRQ), 2011 National Healthcare Disparities Report (NDHR) (Rockville, Md.: AHRQ, 2011).
11. Agency for Healthcare Research and Quality (AHRQ), 2006 National Healthcare Disparities Report (NDHR) (Rockville, Md.: AHRQ, 2006).
12. Frist, William H.(2005). Overcoming Disparities in U.S. Health Care. Health Affairs, 24(2):445-451.
13. McLaughlin, Diane K. , and C. Shannon Stokes,. Income Inequality and Mortality in US Counties: Does Minority Racial Concentration Matter? Am J Public Health. 2002;92:99–104.
14. Henry J. Kaiser Family Foundation (KFF). Key Facts: Race, Ethnicity and Medical Care, 2007 Update. January 2007.
15. Iezzoni, Lisa I. Eliminating Health And Health Care Disparities Among The Growing Population Of People With Disabilities (2011). Health Affairs, 30(10):1947-1954.
16. Probst, Janice C., Jessica D. Bellinger, Katrina M. Walsemann, James Hardin, and Saundra H. Glover (2011). Higher Risk Of Death In Rural Blacks And Whites Than Urbanites Is Related To Lower Incomes, Education, and Health Coverage. Health Affairs 30(10): 1872–1879.
17. Clemans-Cope, Lisa, Genevieve M. Kenney, Matthew Buettgens, Caitlin Carroll and Fredric Blavin (2012). The Affordable Care Act's Coverage Expansions Will Reduce Differences In Uninsurance Rates By Race and Ethnicity. Health Affairs, 31(5):920-930.
18. Biros, Michelle H., James G. Adams, and David C. Cone (2003). Executive Summary: Disparities in Emergency Health Care. Academic Emergency Medicine, 10: 1153–1154.

19. Venkat, A., Hoekstra, J., Lindsell, C., Prall, D., Hollander, J. E., Pollack, C. V., Diercks, D., Kirk, J. D., Tiffany, B., Peacock, F., Storrow, A. B. and Gibler, W. B. (2003). The Impact of Race on the Acute Management of Chest Pain. *Academic Emergency Medicine*, 10: 1199–1208.

20. Bazarian, J. J., Pope, C., McClung, J., Cheng, Y. T. and Flesher, W. (2003). Ethnic and Racial Disparities in Emergency Department Care for Mild Traumatic Brain Injury. *Academic Emergency Medicine*, 10: 1209–1217.

21. O'Connor, R. E. and Haley, L. (2003), Disparities in Emergency Department Health Care: Systems and Administration. *Academic Emergency Medicine*, 10: 1193–1198.

22. Cone, D. C., Richardson, L. D., Todd, K. H., Betancourt, J. R. and Lowe, R. A. (2003). Health Care Disparities in Emergency Medicine. *Academic Emergency Medicine*, 10: 1176–1183.

23. Tamayo-Sarver, J. H., Dawson, N. V., Hinze, S. W., Cydulka, R. K., Wigton, R. S., Albert, J. M., Ibrahim, S. A. and Baker, D. W. (2003). The Effect of Race/Ethnicity and Desirable Social Characteristics on Physicians' Decisions to Prescribe Opioid Analgesics. *Academic Emergency Medicine*, 10: 1239–1248.

24. Cohen, J. J. (2003). Disparities in Health Care: An Overview. *Academic Emergency Medicine*, 10: 1155–1160.

25. Richardson, L. D., Babcock Irvin, C. and Tamayo-Sarver, J. H. (2003). Racial and Ethnic Disparities in the Clinical Practice of Emergency Medicine. *Academic Emergency Medicine*, 10: 1184–1188.

26. Blanchard, J. C., Haywood, Y. C. and Scott, C. (2003). Racial and Ethnic Disparities in Health: An Emergency Medicine Perspective. *Academic Emergency Medicine*, 10: 1289–1293.

27. Marco, Catherine A, Mark Weiner, Sharon L Ream, Dan Lumbrezer, and Djuro Karanovic (2012). Access to care among emergency department patients. *Emergency Medicine Journal*, 29:28e31.

28. Benz, Jennifer K., Oscar Espinosa, Valerie Welsh and Angela Fontes (2011). Awareness Of Racial And Ethnic Health Disparities Has Improved Only Modestly Over A Decade. *Health Affairs*, 30(10):1860-1867.

Chapter 8 References

1. Clemens, M. Kent. "CMS." 1 Estimated Sustainable Growth Rate and Conversion Factor, for Medicare Payments to Physicians in 2011. www.cms.gov/SustainableGRatesConFact/Downloads/sgr2011f.pdf.

2. "2007 Annual Report of the Board of Trustees of the Federal Hospital Insurance and Federal Supplementary Medical Insurance Trust Funds." 2007. Centers for Medicare & Medicaid Services. www.cms.hhs.gov/reportstrustfunds/downloads/tr2007.pdf.

3. COLA. "Medicare and the Sustainable Growth Rate." American Medical Association – Medical Student Section. www.ama-assn.org/ama1/pub/upload/mm/15/cola_medicare_pres.pdf.

4. "Committee on Ways and Means." Hearing Archives. waysandmeans.house.gov/hearings.asp?formmode=view&id=4771.

5. MedPAC. "Report to the Congress: Assessing Alternatives to the Sustainable Growth Rate System." 2007.

6. MedPAC. "Report to the Congress: Medicare Payment Policy." 2008.

7a. MedPAC. "Report to the Congress: Medicare and the Health Care Delivery System." 2012

7. B Congressional Research Service. Medicare Physician Updates and the Sustainable Growth Rate (SGR) System. August 2, 2012. http://usbudgetalert.com/CRS_SGR_Aug%202012.pdf

8. Letter from Congressional Budget Office director Douglas Elmendorf to Senator Harry Reid, December 19, 2009. http://www.cbo.gov/ftpdocs/108xx/doc10868/12-19-Reid_Letter_Managers_Correction_Noted.pdf.

9. Foster RS. Estimated financial effects of the "Patient Protection and Affordable Care Act," as amended. Washington D.C.: Centers for Medicare and Medicaid Services, April 22, 2010.
10. Medicare. http://www.cms.gov/apps/media/press/factsheet.asp?Counter=3823.

Chapter 9 References

1. National Research Council. Best Care at Lower Cost: The Path to Continuously Learning Health Care in America. Washington, DC: The National Academies Press, 2012.
2. Roadmap for Implementing Value Driven Healthcare in the Traditional Medicare Fee-for-Service Program. PDF Document available for download at http://www.cms.gov/QualityInitiativesGenInfo
3. Moody-Williams, J. CMS' Value Based Purchasing: Hospital Value Based Purchasing. Office of Clinical Standards and Quality Centers, Quality Centers for Medicare & Medicaid Services. http://www.hospitalqualityalliance.org.
4. Jencks SF, Williams MV, Coleman EA. Rehospitalizations among patients in the Medicare fee-for-service program. *New England Journal of Medicine*. Apr 2 2009;360(14):1418-1428.
5. Davis, K. Paying for Care Episodes and Care Coordination. *N Engl J Med* 2007; 356: 1166-1168
6. "Bundled Payments for Care Improvement Initiative: Request for Applications." Federal Register 76 (25 Aug 2011): 53137- 53138. http://www.gpo.gov/fdsys/pkg/FR-2011-08-25/pdf/2011-21707.pdf
7. Patient Protection and Affordable Care Act. 2010. Public Law No: 111-148
8. Kaiser Family Foundation. Focus on Health Reform: Summary of New Health Reform Law. www.kff.org/healthreform/upload/8061.pdf
9. Wiler, J. L., D. Beck, et al. (2012). "Episodes of care: is emergency medicine ready?" *Ann Emerg Med.* 59(5): 351-357.
10. ACEP Resolution 17(10): CMS Payment Model Pilot Projects.

Chapter 10 References

1. Centers for Disease Control and Prevention. Emergency Department Visits. http://www.cdc.gov/nchs/fastats/ervisits.htm.
2. Shapiro S, Slone D, et al. Fatal Drug Reactions Among Medical Inpatients. *JAMA*. 1971;216(3):467-472.
3. Ogilvie R, Ruedy J. Adverse drug reactions during hospitalization. *Canad Med Assoc J* 1967:97(24):1450-1457.
4. T.A. Brennan et al., Incidence of Adverse Events and Negligence in Hospitalized Patients. *N Engl J Med* 1991:324(6) 370–376.
5. Leape LL, Bates DW, et al. Systems analysis of adverse drug events. ADE Prevention Study Group. *JAMA*. 1995;274(1):35-43.
6. Institute of Medicine. Crossing the Quality Chasm: A New Health System for the 21st Century. Washington DC: 2001; National Academies Press.
7. Institute of Medicine. The Future of Emergency Care in the United States Health System. Washington, DC: 2006; National Academies Press.
8. Porter ME. What Is Value in Health Care? *N Engl J Med* 2010; 363:2477-2481.
9. Patient Protection and Affordable Care Act. March 23, 2010. P. L. No. 111-148
10. American College of Emergency Physicians. Physician Quality Reporting System FAQ. http://www.acep.org/Content.aspx?id=30492.
11. Centers for Medicare and Medicaid Services. Physician Quality Reporting System. http://www.cms.gov/Medicare/Quality-Initiatives-Patient-Assessment-Instruments/PQRS/index.html?redirect=/pqrs

12. Hospital Outpatient Quality Reporting Program. http://www.qualitynet.org/dcs/ContentSe rver?c=Page&pagename=QnetPublic%2FPage%2FQnetTier3&cid=1192804531207

13. Schuur JD, Brown MD, et al. Assessment of Medicare's Imaging Efficiency Measure for Emergency Department Patients With Atraumatic Headache. *Ann Emerg Med.* 2012;60(3):280–290.

14. Beach C, Croskerry P, Shapiro M. Profiles in Patient Safety: Emergency Care Transitions. *Ann Emerg Med.* 2003;10(4):364–367.

15. Snow V, Beck D, et al. Transitions of Care Consensus Policy Statement: American College of Physicians, Society of General Internal Medicine, Society of Hospital Medicine, American Geriatrics Society, American College of Emergency Physicians, and Society for Academic Emergency Medicine. *J Hosp Med.* 2009;4(6):364–370.

16. American College of Emergency Physicians. *Transitions of Care Task Force Report.* Sept 2012.

17. California Hospital Association. CMS Temporarily Suspends OP-19 for OQR Program. April 4, 2012. http://www.calhospital.org/cha-news-article/cms-temporarily-suspends-op-19-oqr-program

18. Lagu T, Lindenauer, PK. Putting the Public Back in Public Reporting of Healthcare Quality. *JAMA.* 2010;304(15):1711-1712.

19. Chassin MR, Galvin RW, and the National Roundtable on Health Care Quality, The Urgent Need to Improve Health Care Quality. *JAMA.* 1998;280(11):1000–1005.

Chapter 11 References

1. Grumbach, K., & Bodenheimer, T. (2002). A Primary Care Home for Americans. *The Journal of the American Medical Association, 288*(7), 889-893.

2. Landon, B., Gill, J., Antonelli, R., & Rich, E. (2010). Prospects for Rebuilding Primary Care Using the Patient-Centered Medical Home. *Health Affairs, 29*(5), 827-834.

3. Nocon, R., Sharma, R., Birnberg, J., Ngo-Metzger, Q., Lee, S., & Chin, M. (2012). *The Journal of the American Medical Association, 308*(1), 60-66.

4. Crotched Mountain Foundation. *Center for Medical Home Improvement.* Accessed: October, 2012. Retrieved from http://www.medicalhomeimprovement.org.

5. American Academy of Pediatrics. *The National Center for Medical Home Implementation.* Accessed: October, 2012. Retrieved from http://www.medicalhomeinfo.org.

6. American Academy of Family Physicians, American Academy of Pediatrics, American College of Physicians, American Osteopathic Association. (2007). Joint Principles of the Patient-Centered Medical Home. *Patient Cetered Primary Care Collaborative.* Retrieved from http://pcpcc.net.

7. Paulus, R., Davis, K., & Steele, G. (2008). Continuous Innovation in Health Care: Implications of the Geisinger Experience. *Health Affairs, 27*(5), 1235-1245.

8. Community Care of North Carolina. *Community Care of North Carolina: Our Results.* Accessed October, 2012. Retrieved from http://www.communitycarenc.com/our-results.

9. Jaen, C.R., Ferrer, R.L., Miller, W.L., Palmer, R.F., Wood, R., Davila, M., ... Stange, K.C. (2010). Patient outcomes at 26 months in the patient-centered medical home. National Demonstration Project. *Annals of Family Medicine, 8*(4), S57-S67.

10. Flottemesch, T., Anderson, L., Solber, L., Fontaine, P., & Asche, M. (2012). Patient-Centered Medical Home Cost Reductions Limited to Complex Patients. *American Journal of Managed Care, 18(11)*, 677-686.

11. Bitton, A., Martin, C., & Landon, B. (2010). A Nationwide Survey of Patient Centered Medical Home Demonstration Projects. *Journal of General Internal Medicine, 25*(6), 584-592.

12. Reid, R., Fishan, P., Yu, O., Ross, T., Tufano, J., Soman, M., & Larson, E. (2009). Patient-Centered Medical Home Demonstration: A Prospective, Quasi-Experimental, Before and After Evaluation. *American Journal of Managed Care, 15(9)*, e71-87.

13. Department of Health and Human Services, Agency for Healthcare Research and Quality. (2011). Medical Expenditure Panel Survey. Accessed January, 2013. Retrieved from http://meps.ahrq.gov/mepsweb/index.jsp.
14. American College of Emergency Physicians. (2008). *The Patient-Centered Medical Home Model.* Accessed January, 2013. Retrieved from http://www.acep.org/content.aspx?id=42740.
15. Salmon, R.B., Sanderson, M.I., Walters, B.A., Kennedy, K., Flores, R.C., & Muney, A.M. (2012) A collaborative Accountable Care Model in Three Practices Showed Promising Early Results on Costs and Quality of Care. *Health Affairs, 31(11),* 2379-2387.
16. Institute for Health Technology Transformation. (2011). *Accountable Care Organizations: 10 Things You Need to Know About Accountable Care.* Retrieved from http://www.intel.com/content/dam/www/public/us/en/documents/white-papers/10-things-to-know-about-accountable-care-paper.pdf.
17. Mulvany, C. (2011). Medicare ACOs No Longer Mythical Creatures. *Journal of Healthcare Financial Management Association,* 65(6), 96-104.
18. Phillips, R.L., & Bazemore, A. (2010). Primary Care and Why it Matters for U.S. Health System Reform. *Health Affairs,* 29(5), 806-810.
19. Burns, L.R., & Pauly, M.V. (2012). Accountable Care Organizations May Have Difficulty Avoiding the Failures of Integrated Delivery Networks of the 1990's. *Health Affairs,* 31(11), 2407-2416.

Chapter 12 References

1. Emergency Medical Treatment and Active Labor Act, 42 U.S.C. 1395dd
2. American College of Emergency Physicians, *Fact Sheets: Costs of Emergency Care:* http://www3.acep.org/patients.aspx?id=25902, accessed 11/19/2010; American Medical Association Physician Market Place Report: *The Impact of EMTALA on Physicians Practices,* Kane, Carol 5/2003
3. Landmark: The Inside Story of America's New Health Care Law and What It Means for Us All, The Staff of the *Washington Post,* 2010, p 198.
4. Federal Register Vol 75 No 123, June 28, 2010: Rules and Regulations, 37194-5.
5. Federal Register Vol 74 No 123, 37194-5.
6. United States Department of Labor, *Employee Benefits Security Administration: FAQs About the Affordable Care Act Implementation,* http://www.dol.gov/ebsa/faqs/faq-aca.htmlUPICbejB35Y, accessed 1/12/2013.
7. See footnote 7
8. National Association of Insurance Commissioners, *Summary of UCR Senate Hearing Report,* 2009 p1; American Medical News: *United agrees to pay $350 million, scrap system that undercut fees,* http://www.ama-assn.org/amednews/2009/01/26/bil10126.htm, accessed 12/20/2010; Annual Medical Report, *US Senate Commerce Committee Report Criticizes Insurer's Use of Ingenix Inc. Database,* https://www.annualmedicalreport.com/senate-report-criticizes-plans-use-of-ingenix-database/, accessed 01/05/2001; Health Lawyers: *The Ups and Downs of Ingenix UCR Litigation,* Quackenbos, Barbara 2009, http://www.healthlawyers.org/Events/Programs/Materials/Documents/PPMC09/quackenbos.pdf, accessed 01/05/2011 p1.
9. American Medical News: *United agrees to pay $350 million, scrap system that undercut fees,* http://www.ama-assn.org/amednews/2009/01/26/bil10126.htm, accessed 12/20/2010
10. FAIR Health, *About FAIR Health,* http://www.fairhealth.org/about-us, accessed 1/12/2013
11. American Medical News: *FAIR Health database of claims opens to researchers,* http://www.ama-assn.org/amednews/2012/08/06/bise0808.htm, accessed 1/12/2013

12. The New York Times, *Insurers Alter Cost Formula, and Patients Pay More*, Nina Bernstein, http://www.nytimes.com/2012/04/24/nyregion/health-insurers-switch-baseline-for-out-of-network-charges.html?pagewanted=all&_r=0, accessed 1/12/2013

13. Allegany County, State Bills in Progress, http://allegany.ny.networkofcare.org/mh/legislate/state-bill-detail.aspx?bill=A%207489&sessionid=2011000, accessed 10/1/2012

14. *Unexpected Charges: What States Are Doing About Balance Billing*, California HealthCare Foundation Report, April 2009, Hoadley et al.

15. Kaiser Family Foundation, *State Restriction Against Providers Balance Billing Managed Care Enrollees, 2010*, http://www.statehealthfacts.org/comparereport.jsp?rep=66&cat=7, accessed 11/19/2010

16. Hoadley 7

17. Lash 30-31

18. American Medical News, *Model legislation drafted for out-of-network balance billing*, Emily Berry, http://www.ama-assn.org/amednews/2011/03/28/bisd0329.htm, accessed 10/1/2012.

Chapter 13 References

1. Section X: Education and Professional Development – Securing GME Funding for Resident Education. EMRA.org. Accessed 12/22/08

2. CRS Report for Congress. Medicaid and GME funding. http://aging.senate.gov/crs/medicaid8.pdf. Accessed January, 2008.

3. Graduate Medical Education Payments to Teaching Hospitals by Medicare: Unexplained Variation and Public Policy Contradictions. *Acad. Med.* 2001;76:439–445.

4. Report to the Congress: Medicare Payment Policy. March 2010. MedPac. Pp 54 http://www.medpac.gov/documents/Mar10_EntireReport.pdf. accessed August 31, 2010.

5. J. Inglehart, The Uncertain Future of Medicare and Graduate Medical Education, *N Engl J Med* 2011; 365:1340-1345. October, 2011

6. Henderson, T. "Medicaid Direct and Indirect Graduate Medical Education Payments: A 50-State Survey" *AAMC publication*. April, 2010. p 6. Accessed August, 2010

7. Ramano, M. Funding fight. Campaign seeks to boost indirect education payments. *Modern Healthcare*. 2003. Vol. 33 Issue 40, p10.

8. Center for Medicare and Medicaid Services. *Indirect Medical Education (IME)*. http://www.cms.hhs.gov/AcuteInpatientPPS/07_ime.asp#TopOfPage

9. Medicare Indirect Medical Education Payments (IME). http://www.aamc.org/advocacy/library/gme/gme0002.htm.

10. Financing of Emergency Medicine Graduate Medical Education Programs in an Era of Declining Medicare Reimbursement and Support. *Acad Emerg Med* 2004; 11:756–759

11. Medicare payments for Graduate Medical Education: What Every Medical Student, Resident, and Advisor Needs to Know. Association of American Medical Colleges 2006. http://www.uth.tmc.edu/med/administration/gme/pdf_files/medicare_payments_gme.pdf

12 NRMP: Results and Data: Main Residency Match (2012) http://www.nrmp.org/data/resultsanddata2012.pdf

13. NRMP: Results and Data: Main Residency Match (1995) http://www.nrmp.org/data/resultsanddata1995.pdf

14. The Centers for Medicare & Medicaid Services (CMS), inpatient prospective payment system (IPPS) proposed rule for federal fiscal year (FFY) 2013 https://www.cms.gov/Medicare/Medicare-Fee-for-Service-Payment/AcuteInpatientPPS/FY-2013-IPPS-Proposed-Rule-Home-Page.html

15. Williams, E. Public Health, Workforce, Quality, and Related Provisions in the Patient Protection and Affordable Care Act (PPACA). Congressional Research Service. http://www.ncsl.org/documents/health/PHwfQual.pdf. accessed 8/31/10.

16. B. Rye "Assessing the Impact of Potential Cuts in Medicare Doctor-Training Subsidies" 2012 about.bgov.com/bgov/files/2012/03/ryestudy.pdf

17. Securing Medicare GME funding for Outside Rotations. ACEP http://www.acep.org/practres.aspx?id=22488, accessed December 22, 2008.

18. "Public Law 110-252: Making appropriations for military construction, the Department of Veterans Affairs, and related agencies for the fiscal year ending September 30, 2008, and for other purposes." (6/30/08; enacted HR 2642). Text from: United States Public Laws. Available from: The Library of Congress; Accessed: 12/22/08.

19. Thomas Nasca, MD, MACP, et al, "The Potential Impact of Reduction in Federal GME Funding in the United States: A Study of the Estimates of Designated Institutional Officials," http://www.acgme.org/acwebsite/home/ImpactReductionFederalGMEFundingTJN.pdf

20. The Medicare Payment Advisory Commission, *Graduate medical education financing: Focusing on educational priorities* http://www.medpac.gov/chapters/Jun10_Ch04.pdf

21. The National Commission on Fiscal Responsibility and Reform, *The moment of truth: report of the national commission on fiscal responsibility and reform* http://www.fiscalcommission.gov/sites/fiscalcommission.gov/files/documents/TheMomentofTruth12_1_2010.pdf

22. The Congressional Budget Office, *choices for deficit reduction* http://www.cbo.gov/sites/default/files/cbofiles/attachments/43692-DeficitReduction_print.pdf

23. AAMC Washington Highlights. "AAMC Applauds the Reintroduction of House and Senate GME Bills" March 15, 2013. https://www.aamc.org/advocacy/washhigh/highlights2013/331020/031513aamcapplaudsthereintroductionofhouseandsenategmebills.html.

Chapter 14 References

1. Databases, Tables & Calculators by Subject." U.S. Bureau of Labor Statistics. Web. July 2010. http://www.bls.gov/data.

2. Federal Student Aid, An Office of the U.S. Department of Education. Web. Dec 2012. http://studentaid.ed.gov/types/loans/subsidized-unsubsidized

3. "Graduate Stafford Student Loan – Graduate Federal Stafford Loans for Graduate School." Graduate Loans – Financial Aid for Grad School. StudentLoanNetwork. Web. July 2010. http://www.gradloans.com/stafford_loan.

4. "Funding Education Beyond High School: The Guide to Federal Student Aid 2009-10." FSA Portals. Federal Student Aid. Web. July 2010. http://studentaid.ed.gov/students/publications/student_guide/2009-2010/english/postponeloanpayment.htm.

5. "The 20/220 Pathway and Income Based Repayment." American Medical Association. *AMA*, July 2010. Web. http://www.ama-assn.org/ama/pub/about-ama/our-people/member-groups-sections/medical-student-section/advocacy-policy/medical-student-debt/20-220-pathway-ibr.shtml.

6. "National Health Service Corps." National Health Service Corps HRSA. Web. July 2010.

7. Slack, Megan. "Income Based Repayment: Everything You Need to Know" The White House. 7 June 2012. Web Oct. 2012.http://www.whitehouse.gov/the-press-office/2011/10/25/fact-sheet-help-americans-manage-student-loan-debt

8. Eli, Adashi, MD, MS Y., and Gruppuso, MD A. Philip. "Commentary: The Unsustainable Cost of Undergraduate Medical Education: An Overlooked Element of the U.S. Health Care Reform." *Academic Medicine* 85.5: 763-5. PubMed. July 2010. Web. 8 July 2010. http://www.ncbi.nlm.nih.gov/pubmed.

9. "AAMC Survey of Resident/Fellow Stipends and Benefits." AAMC. AAMC, July 2010. Web. 8 July 2010. http://www.aamc.org/data/stipend/2009_stipendreport.pdf.

10. "Physician Specialty Databook 2012" AAMC. Web. Dec 2012. https://members.aamc.org/
eweb/DynamicPage.aspx?Action=Add&ObjectKeyFrom=1A83491A-9853-4C87-86A4-F7
D95601C2E2&WebCode=PubDetailAdd&DoNotSave=yes&ParentObject=CentralizedOrd
erEntry&ParentDataObject=Invoice%20Detail&ivd_formkey=69202792-63d7-4ba2-bf4e-
a0da41270555&ivd_prc_prd_key=C7F68470-F2D7-45AA-BC1D-DB67C3F2D318.

Chapter 15 References

1. Council on Graduate Medical Education. 2005. *Physician Workforce Policy Guidelines for the United States, 2000-2020.* Sixteenth Report. Rockville, MD: U.S. Department of Health and Human Services.

2. Camargo, Jr., CA, AA Ginde, AH Singer, JA Espinola, AF Sullivan, JF Pearson, and AJ Singer. 2008. Assessment of Emergency Physician Workforce Needs in the United States, 2005. *Academic Emergency Medicine* 15(12): 1317-1320.

2.5 Association of American Medical Colleges Center for Workforce Studies. Recent studies and reports on physician shortages in the US. October 2012.

3. Bureau of Health Professions. 2006. *Physician Supply and Demand: Projections to 2020.* Washington, DC: U.S. Department of Health and Human Services.

4. Owens, P *et al.* 2010. Emergency department care in the United States: A profile of national data sources. *Annals of Emergency Medicine* 56(2):150-65.

5. Tang, N, J Stein, R Hsia, J Maselli, R Gonzalez. 2010. Trends and characteristics of US emergency department visits, 1997-2007. *JAMA* 304(6):664-70.

6. CDC. Emergency Department Visits (2011). Available online at: http://www.cdc.gov/nchs/fastats/ervisits.htm (Accessed October, 2012)

7. Sullivan *et al.* 2009. Supply and demand of board-certified emergency physicians by US state, 2005. *Academic Emergency Medicine* 16(10):1014-18.

8. Ginde A, A Sullivan, C Camargo. 2009. National study of the emergency physician workforce, 2008. *Annals of Emergency Medicine* 54(3):349-58.

9. Ginde, A *et al.* 2010. Attrition from emergency medicine clinical practice in the United States. *Annals of Emergency Medicine* 56(2):166-71. Handel, D, J Hedges. 2007. Improving rural access to emergency physicians. *Academic Emergency Medicine* 14(6):562-65.

10. Institute of Medicine of the National Academies. 2006. Future of Emergency Care Series: Hospital-Based Emergency Care At the Breaking Point. Washington, DC: National Academy Press.

11. Schneider, S *et al.* 2010. The future of Emergency Medicine. *Annals of Emergency Medicine* 56(2):178-83.

12. Rao MB, Lerro C, Gross CP. The shortage of on-call surgical specialist coverage: a national survey of emergency department directors. *Acad Emerg Med.* 2010 Dec;17(12):1374-82.

13. Rudkin SE, Langdorf MI, Oman JA, et, al. The worsening of ED on-call coverage in California: 6-year trend. *Am J Emerg Med.* 2009 Sep;27(7):785-91.

14. Bodenheimer, T, RA Berenson, and P Rudolf. 2007. The Primary Care-Specialty Income Gap: Why it Matters. *Annals of Internal Medicine* 146(4): 301-6.

154. Council on Graduate Medical Education. 1998. *Physician Distribution and Health Care Challenges in Rural and Inner-City Areas.* Tenth Report. Rockville, MD: U.S. Department of Health and Human Services.

16. Ginde AA, Rao M, Simon EL, et, al. Regionalization of emergency care future directions and research: workforce issues. *Acad Emerg Med.* 2010 Dec;17(12):1286-96.

17. Handel , DA, JR Hedges 2007. Improving rural access to emergency physicians. *Academic Emergency Medicine* 14:562-565.

18. Long SK, Phadera L. 2010. *Barriers to obtaining health care among insured Massachusetts residents.* Rep. Mass. Div. Health Care Finance and Policy, May. http://www.mass.gov/Eeohhs2/docs/dhcfp/r/pubs/10/barriers_policy_brief_2010_05.pdf

19. Kirch DG, Henderson MK, Dill MJ. Physician workforce projections in an era of health care reform. *Annu Rev Med.* 2012;63:435-45.
20. Katz, M. 2010. Future of the safety net under health reform. *JAMA* 304(6):679-80.
21. Arvantes J. Provisions in health care reform law lay out role of primary care, family physicians: measures place greater emphasis on prevention, care coordination. http://www.aafp.org/online/en/home/publications/news/news-now/government-medicine/20100728hcreformoverview.html. July, 2010.
22. ACEP Strategic Plan, 2010-2013.
23. AAMC. "Medical School Enrollment Continues to Climb with New Diversity Gains: New Residency Positions Needed for M.D.s to Complete Training. Available online at: https://www.aamc.org/newsroom/newsreleases/310002/121023.html (Accessed January, 2013)
24. Council on Graduate Medical Education. 2007. *Enhancing Flexibility in Graduate Medical Education.* Nineteeth Report. Rockville, MD: U.S. Department of Health and Human Services.
25. Ginsburg, P, and RA Berenson. 2007. Revising Medicare's Physician Fee Schedule—Much Activity, Little Change. *New England Journal of Medicine* 356(12): 1201-1203.
26. Lasser, KE, S Woolhandler, and DU Himmelstein. 2008. Sources of U.S. Physician Income: The Contribution of Government Payments to the Specialist-Generalist Income Gap. *Journal of General Internal Medicine* 23(9): 1477-81.
27. Powers, R. 2000. Emergency Department Use by Adult Medicaid Patients after Implementation of Managed Care. *Academic Emergency Medicine* 7(12): 1416-20.
28. National Advisory Committee on Rural Health and Human Services. 2008. The 2008 Report to the Secretary: Rural Health and Human Services Issues. U.S. Department of Health and Human Services.
29. ACEP Academic Affairs Committee. "Medical Education Debt/Loan Reapyment-Forgiveness." Available online at: http://www.acep.org/content.aspx?id=22472 (Accessed January, 2013)
30. Tally BE, Ann Moore S, Camargo CA Jr., et, al. Availability and potential effect of rural rotations in emergency medicine residency programs. *Acad Emerg Med.* 2011 Mar;18(3):297-300.
31. Wadman MC, Fago B, Hoffman, et, al. A comparison of emergency medicine resident clinical experience in a rural versus urban emergency department. *Rural Remote Health.* 2010 Apr-Jun;10(2):1442.
32. *Acad Emerg Med.* 2010 Dec;17(12):1286-96. doi: 10.1111/j.1553-2712.2010.00938. xRao MB, Lerro C, Gross CP. *Acad Emerg Med.* 2010 Dec;17(12):1374-82. doi: 10.1111/j.1553-2712.2010.00927.x. Epub 2010 Nov. Menchine MD, Baraff LJ. *Acad Emerg Med.* 2008 Apr;15(4):329-36. *Am J Emerg Med.* 2009 Sep;27(7):785-91. Hooker RS, Klocko DJ, Larkin GL. Physician assistants in emergency medicine: the impact of their role. *Acad Emerg Med.* 2011 Jan;18(1):72-7.

Chapter 16 References

1. Rao MB, Lerro C, Gross C. The Shortage of On-call Surgical Specialist Coverage: A National Survey of Emergency Department Directors. *Acad Emerg Med.* 2010;17(12):1374–1382.
2. Cafee H, Rudnick C. Access to Hand Surgery Emergency Care. *Ann Plast Surg.* 2007; 58:207-208.
3. Rudkin SE, Oman J, Langdorf MI, et al. The States of Emergency Department on-call Coverage in California. *Am J Emerg Med.* 2004; 22(7):575-581.
4. Medicare Program: Clarifying Policies Related to the Responsibilities of Medicare Participating Hospitals in Treating Individuals with Emergency Medical Conditions. Final Rule. *Fed Regist.* 2003 Sep 9; 68(174):53222-64.
5. Center for Studying Health Systems Change. Hospital Emergency On-call Coverage: Is There a Doctor in the House? http://www/hschange.org/
6. Fosmire S. EMTALA FAQ, 2009. http://emtala.com/faq.org
7. Fosmire S. EMTALA FAQ, 2009. http://emtala.com/faq.org
8. Fosmire S. EMTALA FAQ, 2009. http://emtala.com/faq.org
9. Inpatient Prospective Payment System (IPPS) 2009 Final Rule Revisions to Emergency Medical Treatment and Labor Act (EMTALA) Regulations. Centers for Medicare and Medicaid Services: Department of Health and Human Services, March 2009. http://www.gpo.gov/fdsys/pkg/FR-2012-02-02/html/2012-2287.htm
10. McConnell KJ, Johnson LA, Arab N, et al. The on-call crisis: A statewide assessment of the costs of providing on-call specialist coverage. *Ann Emerg Med.* 2007;49(6):727-733,e721-718.
11. Regionalizing Emergency Care: Workshop Summary. Institute of Medicine Washington, DC: national Academies Press. 2010. http://www.iom.edu
12. Hansel P. California Senate Office of Research. Stretched Thin: Growing Gaps in California's Emergency room Backup System. California Senate Office of Research, 2003. http://cdm16254.contentdm.oclc.org/cdm/singleitem/collection/p17860lccp2/id/3095/rec/10
13. SEC. 5000A: Requirement to Maintain Essential Coverage. The Patient Protection and Affordable Care Act. Ppaca&Hcera; PublicLaws 111-148 & 111-152: Consolidated Print. January 2010.
14. Garcia TC, Bernstein AB, and Bush MA. Emergency Department Visitors and Visits: Who Used the Emergency Room in 2007? *NCHS Data Brief*, No. 38, May 2010. http://www.cdc.gov/nchs/data/databriefs/db38.pdf
15. Tang N, Stein J, Hsia R, Maselli J, Gonzales R. Trends and Characteristics of US Emergency Department Visits, 1997-2007. JAMA, August. 2010; 304(6): 664–670. doi: 10.1001/jama.2010.1112
16. Patient Health Safety Act, Title 42 USCA§300gg-19a, Section 2719A
17. H.R. 1188–111th Congress: Access to Emergency Medical Services Act of 2009. http://www.govtrack.us/congress/bills/111/hr118 (HR 3875 in 2005, HR 882 in 2007)
18. Zibulewsky, J. The Emergency Medical Treatment and Active Labor Act (EMTALA): what it is and what it means for physicians. Proc (Bayl Univ Med Cent). October 2001; 14(4): 339–346.
19. Zibulewsky, J. The Emergency Medical Treatment and Active Labor Act (EMTALA): what it is and what it means for physicians. Proc (Bayl Univ Med Cent). October 2001; 14(4): 339–346.
20. Rules of Department of Health and Senior Services. Division of Regulation and Licensure. 19 CSR 30-20.092. October 2011. http://www.sos.mo.gov/adrules/csr/current/19csr/19c30-20.pdf
21. 45 N.J. Reg. 8:43G-5.1 (November 2008) (Administrative and hospital-wide structural organization).

22. 45 N.J. Reg. 8:43G-12.5 (April 2002) (Emergency department staff time and availability).
23. The Impact of Health Care Reform on the Future Supply and Demand for Physicians Updated Projections Through 2025., AAMC. June 2010. https://www.aamc.org/download/158076/data/updated_projections_through_2025.pdf
24. Harris S. Physician Shortage Spreads Across Specialty Lines. AAMC. October 2010. https://www.aamc.org/newsroom/reporter/oct10/152090/physician_shortage_spreads_across_specialty_lines.html
25. Darves, B. Physician Shortages in the Specialties Taking a Toll. Effects of the increasing undersupply are palpable in recruiting, not just patient-access difficulties. *New England Journal of Medicine*, Career Center. March 2011.
26. A growing crisis in patient access to emergency surgical care. The American College of Surgeons, Division of Health Advocacy and Health Policy. *Bull Am Coll Surg*. August 2006;91(8):8-19. www.facs.org/ahp/emergcarecrisis.pdf
27. 2011 Physician Retention Survey, Cejka Search and AMGA, March 12. http://www.cejkasearch.com/news/press-releases/physician-shortage-challenges-medical-groups-and-increases-demand-for-advanced-practitioners
28. American College of Surgeons. FAQ for Resources for Optimal Care for the Injured Patient. http://www/facs.org/trauma/faq_answers.html
29 Rao MB, Lerro C, Gross C. The Shortage of On-call Surgical Specialist Coverage: A National Survey of Emergency Department Directors. *Acad Emerg Med*. 2010;17(12):1374–1382.
30. Vanlandingham B. On-call Specialist Coverage in the U.S. Emergency Departments, Irving TX: American College of Emergency Physicians. 2004.
31. DiRosa R, Brennan G, D'Souza I, Houchins-Witt C, Smith M. United States General Accounting Office. Medical malpractice: Implications of rising premiums and access to healthcare. August 2003. http://www.gao.gov/new.items/d03836.pdf
32. Hsia R, Shen Y.Changes in Geographical Access to Trauma Centers for Vulnerable Populations in the United States. Health Aff (Millwood). October 2011; 30(10): 1912–1920.
33. AAMC Center for Workforce Studies. From ACA. Sec. 1281. https://www.aamc.org/download/124782/data/healthcarereform.pdf
34. EMTALA, Section 1866 (a)(1): CMS does not have requirements regarding how frequently on call physicians are expected to be available to provide on call coverage. Nor is there a pre-determined ratio CMS uses to identify how many days a hospital must provide medical staff on-call coverage. On-call coverage is a decision made by hospital administrators and the physicians who provide on-call coverage for the hospital. The list cannot be physician group names, must be individual provider name.
35. Zibulewsky, J. The Emergency Medical Treatment and Active Labor Act (EMTALA): what it is and what it means for physicians. Proc (Bayl Univ Med Cent). October 2001; 14(4): 339–346.
36. Rules of Department of Health and Senior Services . Division of Regulation and Licensure. 19 CSR 30-20.092. October 2011. http://www.sos.mo.gov/adrules/csr/current/19csr/19c30-20.pdf
37. 8:43G-5.1 Administrative and hospital-wide structural organization, NJ ADC 8:43G-5.1 January, 2013; 45 N.J. Reg. No. 1
38. 8:43G-12.5 Emergency department staff time and availability, NJ ADC 8:43G-12.5. January, 2013; 45 N.J. Reg. No. 1
39. EA Health. On-call Compensation. EA Health Company website. http://www.eahealth.co/services/on-call-compensation
40. Taylor T. Innovative Solutions to On-Call ED Specialty Coverage and Ensuring Adequate On-Call Backup in the ED. Interim AMA Organized Medical Staff Section Assembly, *ACEP Clinical and Practice Management 2005*. www.acep.org/workarea/downloadasset.aspx?id=37944

41. H.R. 3875–109th Congress: Access to Emergency Medical Services Act of 2005. (2005). http://www.govtrack.us/congress/bills/109/hr3875
42. Physician Assistants. Bureau of Labor Statistics, U.S. Department of Labor, Occupational Outlook Handbook, 2012-13. http://www.bls.gov/ooh/healthcare/physician-assistants.htm
43. The Physician Assistant History Society, Inc. http://www.pahx.org/period08.html
44 Fosmire S. EMTALA FAQ, 2009. http://emtala.com/faq.org
45 McAneny B. Emergency Room Contracts and Hospital Privileges: Executive Summary: Report 1 of the Council on Medical Service. I-09; Resolution 806, I-08. http://www.ama-assn.org/resources/doc/cms/i09-cms-report1.pdf.

Chapter 17 References

1. AMA FREIDA Specialty Training Data. https://freida.ama-assn.org/Freida/user/specStatisticsSearch.do?method=viewDetail&spcCd=110&pageNumber=2
2. ABEM Certification Data – 12/31/2009. https://www.abem.org
3. BUIE, Louis. Specialty Certifying Boards in American Medicine. *British Medical Journal.* 1965, 1, 543-547. http://www.ncbi.nlm.nih.gov/pmc/articles/PMC2166804/pdf/brmedj02383-0027.pdf
4. ABMS History. http://www.abms.org/About_ABMS/ABMS_History/Extended_History/Becoming_ABMS.aspx
5. ABEM History. https://www.abem.org/PUBLIC/portal/alias__Rainbow/lang__en-US/tabID__3573/DesktopDefault.aspx
6. Appellate Decision in Second Circuit Court. http://www.ca2.uscourts.gov
7. ABPS – About Us. http://www.abpsus.org/about-abps
8. Florida Board of Medicine. https://www.flrules.org/gateway/RuleNo.asp?title=ADVERTISING&ID=64B8-11.001
9. Appellate Decision in Second Circuit Court. http://www.ca2.uscourts.gov/decisions/isysquery/b2a1537f-f212-4804-8d1c-451f40ef30fb/1/doc/09-4325_so.pdf#xml=http://www.ca2.uscourts.gov/decisions/isysquery/b2a1537f-f212-4804-8d1c-451f40ef30fb/1/hilite
10. Ayres, Ronald E; S Scheinthal, C Gross, and E Bell. "Changes to Osteopathic Specialty Board Certification." *Journal of the American Osteopathic Association* 112 (4): 226-231.

Chapter 18 References

1. Schneider et al. The Future of Emergency Medicine. *Acad Em Med.* 2010:17(9): 998–1003
2. Lane S, Scott C. Twenty-Sixth Annual Report on Physician Assistant Educational Programs in the United States, 2009-2010. Physician Assistant Education Association; January 2012.
3. SEMPA. Becoming an EMPA. Visited 2/10/13. http://www.sempa.org/becoming-an-empa
4. American Academy of Physician Assistants. (2011). 2010 AAPA Physician Assistant Census. Alexandria, VA.
5. Arbet et al. Report on Emergency Medicine Physician's Assistants. 2009.
6. Competencies for the Physician Assistant Profession.Physican Assistant Education Association. Visited 08/14/12, http://www.paeaonline.org/index.php?ht=a/GetDocumentAction/i/113465
7. NCCPA. Emergency Medicine CAQ. Visited 2/10/2013, http://www.nccpa.net/Emergencymedicine.aspx#introduction
8. http://www.mdapa.org/maryland/differences.asp
9. Nurse Practitioner/Advanced Practice Nursing Network Policy Statement. Definition and characteristics of the role. Visited on 9/11/12. http://icn-apnetwork.org

10. National Organization of Nurse Practitioner Faculties.Nurse Practitioner Core Competencies. Visited 9/11/12, http://www.nonpf.com/associations/10789/files/ NPCoreCompetenciesFinal2012.pdf

11. National Organization of Nurse Practitioner Faculties. Nurse Practitioner Core Competencies. Visited 9/11/12, http://www.nonpf.com/associations/10789/files/ NPCoreCompetenciesFinal2012.pdf

12. Emory University Emergency Nurse Practitioner Fellowship Program Overview. Visited 7/7/12, http://www.nursing.emory.edu/admission/masters/specialties/emergency_ np.html

13. Camargo CA Jr et al. Assessment of emergency physician workforce needs in the United States, 2005. Acad Emerg Med. 2008 Dec;15(12):1317-20. Epub Oct 2008.

14. Fronstin, P. The The impact of the recession on employment-based health coverage. EBRI Issue Brief. 2010 May;(342):1-22.

15. Schneider et al. The Future of Emergency Medicine. Acad Em Med. 2010:17(9): 998–1003

16. Menchine MD, Weichmann W, Rudkin S. Trends in midlevel provider utilization in emergency departments from 1997 to 2006. Acad Emerg Med. 2009;16(10):963-969

17. U.S. General Accounting Office. Nursing Workforce: Emerging Nurse Shortages Due to Multiple Factors. Washington DC: US General Accounting Office, July 2001. http://www. gao.gov/new.items/d01944.pdf.

18. Arbet et al. Report on Emergency Medicine Physician's Assistants. 2009.

19. Schneider et al. The Future of Emergency Medicine. Acad Em Med. 2010:17(9): 998–1003

20. Advance Magazine 2011 Physician Assistant Salary Report. Visited 9/10/12, http://nurse-practitioners-and-physician-assistants.advanceweb.com/Web-Extras/Online-Extras/2011-NP-PA-Salary-Survey-Results.aspx

21. Advance Magazine 2011 Nurse Practitioner Salary Report. Visited 9/10/12, http://nurse-practitioners-and-physician-assistants.advanceweb.com/SignUp/ RegDocFetchFile.aspx?BRID=2163138281E77

22. Medscape 2012 Emergency Medicine Physician compensation report. Visited 9/11/12, http://www.medscape.com/features/slideshow/compensation/2012/emergencymedicine

23. Ppaca&Hcera;PublicLaws111-148&111-152: ConsolidatedPrint. http://www.ncsl.org/ documents/health/ppaca-consolidated.pdf

24. Gind, AA et al. Am J Emerg Med 2010;28[1]:90.

25. Arbet et al. Report on Emergency Medicine Physician's Assistants. 2009.

26. Am J Emerg Med 2010;28[4]:485

27. Emergency Medicine Residency Association. Policy Compendium. Section X, Part XXXII Role of Physician Extenders in Emergency Medicine, 2010. http://www.emra.org/ uploadedFiles/EMRA/About_EMRA/Governing_Documents/Policy_Compendium(1).pdf

28. Brown et al. Continued rise in the use of midlevel providers in US emergency departments, 1993-2009. Int J Emerg Med. 2012 May 23;5(1):21.

29. AAEM Policy statement http://www.aaem.org/em-resources/position-statements/2000/ physician-asst

30. ACEP Policy Statements. Guidelines Regarding the Role of Physician Assistants and Nurse Practicioners in the Emergency Department. 2007.

31. Quynh, D et al. A systematic review: The role and impact of the physician assistant in the emergency department. Emergency Medicine Australia. Volume 23, Issue 1. Feb 2011.

32. Elliott EP, Erdman K, Waters V et al. Opinions of Texas emergency medicine physicians regarding the use of physician assistants in the emergency department. J. Physician Assist. Educ. 2007; 18 (4):40–3.

33. CopIan B, Richardson L, Stoehr J. Physician assistant program medical directors' opinions of an entry-level physician assistant clinical doctorate degree. J Phys Assist Educ. 2009;20(2):8-13.

34. Patient perceptions regarding health care providers. *AAFP Publication.* http://www.aafp.
org/online/etc/medialib/aafp_org/documents/membership/nps/perceptions.Par.0001.
File.tmp/PatientPerceptions.pdf

35. American Association of Colleges of Nursing. DNP Roadmap Task Force Report 2006.
http://www.aacn.nche.edu/dnp/pdf/DNProadmapreport.pdf

36. Marion L, Viens D, O'Sullivan AL, Crabtree K, Fontana S, Price MM. The practice
doctorate in nursing: Future or fringe? *Top Adv Pract Nursing E-Journal.* 2003;3(2).
http:// www.medscape.com/viewarticle/453247

37. American Medical Association. Resolution. 211(A-06) Need to expose and counter nurse
doctoral programs misrepresentation. http://www.ama-assn.org

Chapter 19 References

1. Chamberlain LJ, Sanders LM, Takayama JI. Child advocacy training: curriculum outcomes
and resident satisfaction. *Arch Pediatr Adolesc Med.* 2005;159(9):842-7.

2. Accreditation Council for Graduate Medical Education. Pediatrics program requirements.
http://www.acgme.org/acWebsite/RRC_320/320_prIndex.asp.

3. Earnest MA, Wong SL, Federico SG. Perspective: Physician advocacy: what is it and how do
we do it? *Acad Med.* 2010;85(1):63-7.

4. Code of ethics for emergency physicians. *Ann Emerg Med.* 2008;52(5):581-90. http://
www.acep.org/Clinical---Practice-Management/Code-of-Ethics-for-Emergency-
Physicians.

5. Ptakowski KK. Advocating for children and adolescents with mental illnesses. *Child Adolesc
Psychiatr Clin N Am.* 2010;19(1):131-8; table of contents.

6. Hurley KF. Advocacy and activism in emergency medicine. *CJEM.* 2007;9(4):282-5.

7. Fisher H, Drummond A. A call to arms: The emergency physician, international
perspectives on firearm injury prevention and the Canadian gun control debate. *J Emerg
Med.* 1999;17(3):529-37.

8. Lai J. Health advocacy in emergency medicine: A resident's perspective. *CJEM.*
2009;11(1):99-100.

9. Christoffel KK. Public health advocacy: Process and product. *Am J Public Health.*
2000;90(5):722-6.

10. Asplin BR, Knopp RK. A room with a view: On-call specialist panels and other health policy
challenges in the emergency department. *Ann Emerg Med.* 2001;37(5):500-3.

11. Landers SH, Sehgal AR. How do physicians lobby their members of Congress? *Arch Intern
Med.* 2000;160(21):3248-51.

12. Kane C. *American Medical Association Physician Marketplace Report: The Impact of
EMTALA on Physician Practices.* Feb. 2003. www.ama-assn.org/resources/doc/health-
policy/pmr2003-02.pdf

13. Hemphill RR, et al. Emergency medicine and political influence. *Acad Emerg Med.*
2009;16(10):1019-24.

14. Kush C. *The One-Hour Activist: The 15 Most Powerful Actions You Can Take to Fight for
the Issues and Candidates You Care About.* San Francisco: Jossey-Bass; 2004.

15. Newman TB. The power of stories over statistics. *BMJ.* 2003;327(7429):1424-7.

16. Stokowski LA, et al. Advocacy: It is what we do. *Adv Neonatal Care.* 2010;10(2):75-82.

17. Kraus JF, Fife D, Conroy C. Incidence, severity, and outcomes of brain injuries involving
bicycles. *Am J Public Health.* 1987;77(1):76-8.

18. Thompson RA, Et al. A case-control study of the effectiveness of bicycle safety helmets.
N Engl J Med. 1989;320:1361-1367.

19. Peters JW. Obama Looks to Expand Campaign's Reach Through Social Media. *New York
Times.* March 14, 2012. http://www.nytimes.com/2012/03/15/us/politics.

20. Fox News. *Political parties use social media to open up convention process.* http://soc.li/YscnWFe.
21. Cohen CJ, Kahne J. *Participatory politics: New media and youth political action.* MacArthur Research Network on Youth and Participatory Politics. 2012. ypp.dmlcentral.net
22. Huddle TS. Perspective: Medical professionalism and medical education should not involve commitments to political advocacy. *Acad Med.* 2011;86(3):378-83.
23. Glassick CE. Boyer's expanded definitions of scholarship, the standards for assessing scholarship, and the elusiveness of the scholarship of teaching. *Acad Med.* 2000; 75(9): 877-80.

Chapter 20 References

1. School House Rock. "I'm Just a Bill" http://www.schoolhouserock.tv/Bill.html. Accessed December, 2012.
2. United States House of Representatives: http://www.house.gov. Accessed December, 2012.
3. United States Senate: http://senate.gov. Accessed December, 2012.
4. The United States Senate Committee on Finance. "Health Care Reform from Conception to Final Passage." Accessed December, 2012.
5. "Roll call vote No. 887: On Passage of the Affordable Health Care for America Act." Office of the Clerk: House of Representatives. Accessed December, 2012.
6. "Roll Call vote No. 396: On Passage of the Bill (H.R. 3590 as Amended)." U.S. Senate. Accessed December, 2012.
7. "Roll Call vote No. 165: On Motion to Concur in Senate Amendments (Patient Protection and Affordable Care Act)." Office of the Clerk: House of Representatives. Accessed December, 2012.
8. Supreme Court of the United States. www.supremecourt.gov. Accessed December, 2012.
9. United States House of Representatives: http://www.house.gov. Accessed December, 2012

Chapter 22 References

1. American College of Emergency Physicians. *Advocacy.* Building a Coalition. http://www.acept.org/ACEP-Taxonomy-of-Subject-Matterews-/Building-a-Coalition
2. *Collins English Dictionary - Complete & Unabridged 10th Edition.* Coalition. HarperCollins Publishers. Dictionary.com http://dictionary.reference.com/browse/coalition
3. *Dictionary.com's 21st Century Lexicon.* Dictionary.com, LLC. Coalition Government. Dictionary.com http://dictionary.reference.com/browse/coalition government
4. Mitchner J, et al. Building Successful Coalitions. Physicians' Guide to State Legislation. 3rd ed. Dallas: ACEP, 1997. 46-49.
5. American Medical Association. Our Mission. http://www.ama-assn.org/ama/pub/about-ama/our-mission
6. Protect Patients Now. Who We Are. http://www.hcla.org/content/who-we-are.
7. Washington Academy of Family Physicians. WSHA, WSMA, & ACEP Team Up to address ED Overuse Debate. Bellevue, June 2012. http://wafp.net/News/News/WSHA,-WSMA---ACEP-Team-Up-to-a.aspx

Chapter 23 References

1. Schneider ME. Legislating Medicine State by State. *ACEP News.* August, 2012.
2. Grill C. Navigating the Legislative Process. *Bull Am Coll Surg.* 2011; 96(4):44-5, 60.
3. Hemphill RR, Sklar DP, Christopher T, Kellerman AL, Tarrant JR. Emergency Medicine and Political Influence. *Acad Emerg Med.* 2009; 16:1019-24.
4. Code of Ethics for Emergency Physicians. American College of Emergency Physicians. 2001. Available: http://www.acep.org.
5. Collins, J. Good to Great. 2001. HarperCollins Publishers, Inc. New York, NY.
6. Hurley KF. Advocacy and Activism in Emergency Medicine. *Can J Emerg Med.* 2007; 9(4):283-5.
7. Newman, TM. The Power of Stories over Statistics. *BMJ.* 2003; 327:1424-7.
8. Collins, M. States Enact Liability Reforms Specific to Emergency Care. *ACEP Clinical and Practice Management.* 2008. Available: www.acep.org.
9. Darves B. Texas Tort Reform: One Year Later, Some Physicians Say They're Reaping Big Benefits. *ACP Internist.* 2005. Available: www.acpinternist.org.
10. Hoyer D. Tort Reform Shows Positive Results in TX and CA. *Emergency Physicians Monthly.* 2010. Available: www.epmonthly.com.
11. Katz G. Personal Communication. September 13, 2012.

Chapter 24 References

1. Agency for Healthcare Research and Quality. "What is AHRQ?" Available at http://archive.ahrq.gov/about/whatis.htm. Accessed September, 2012
2. "The Health Insurance Experiment: A Classic RAND Study Speaks to the Current Health Reform Debate." RAND Corporation. http://www.rand.org/content/dam/rand/pubs/research_briefs/2006/RAND_RB9174.pdf. Accessed September, 2012.
3. Concato J. Is It Time for Medicine-Based Evidence? *JAMA.* 2012 Apr 18;307(15):1641-3.
4. Kocher KE, Meurer WJ, Desmond JS, Nallamothu BK. Effect of testing and treatment on emergency department length of stay using a national database. *Acad Emerg Med.* 2012 May;19(5):525-34.
5. Wiler JL, Rooks SP, Ginde AA. Update on midlevel provider utilization in U.S. emergency departments, 2006 to 2009. *Acad Emerg Med.* 2012 Aug;19(8):986-9.
6. Venkatesh AK, Geisler BP, Gibson Chambers JJ, Baugh CW, Bohan JS, Schuur JD. Use of observation care in US emergency departments, 2001 to 2008. *PLoS One.* 2011;6(9):e24326.

Chapter 25 References

1. Studdert, D., "RAND Review: Patching holes in the medical malpractice system is no longer enough." Summer 2004. http://www.rand.org/publications/randreview/issues/summer2004/35.html. Accessed September, 2010.
2. Anderson, R., "Commentaries Defending the Practice of Medicine." *Archive of Internal Medicine.* June 14, 2004. 164: 1173-4
3. Noneconomic Damages Reform. *American tort Reform Association.* http://www.atra.org/issues/noneconomic-damages-reform. Accessed January, 2013.
4. Mello, M. , Studdert, D., DesRoches, C. , et al. "Effects of a Malpractice Crisis on Specialist Supply and Patient Access to Care." *Ann Surg.* 2005 November; 242(5): 621–628.
5. First Professionals Insurance Company. 2007. PIAA Claim Trend Analysis: 2006 ed.
6. Studdertt DM, Mello M, Gawande AA, Gandhi TK, Kachalia A, Yoon C, Puopolo AL, Brennan TA. Claims, errors, and compensation payments in medical malpractice litigation. *N. Eng J. Med.* May 11, 2006; 354(19):2024-33

7. Studdert DM, Mello MM, Sage WM, DesRoches CM, Peugh J, Zapert K, Brennan TA. "Defensive medicine among high-risk specialist physicians in a volatile malpractice environment." *JAMA*. 2005 Jun 1; 293(21):2660-2.
8. American Medical Association. Medical Liability Reform – NOW! February, 2008. http://www.ama-assn.org/ama1/pub/upload/mm/-1/mlrnow.pdf. Accessed September, 2010.
9. American College of Emergency Physicians. Reform of Tort Law Policy Statement. August 2009. http://www.acep.org/practres.aspx?id=29666. Accessed September, 2010.
10. Weiss LD, Li J. AAEM White Paper on Tort Reform. A policy Paper of the American Academy of Emergency Medicine. *J Emerg Med*. 2006; 30473-475.
11. American Tort Reform Association, ATRA Tort Reform Record. July 2010. http://www.atra.org/files.cgi/8496_record_7-1-10.pdf. Accessed September, 2010.
12. Bernstein, J., MacCourt, D., Abramson, B., "Topics in Medical Economics: Medical Malpractice." *J Bone Joint Surg Am*. 2008;90:1777-82
13. Letourneau R., "Defensive Medicine Adds Billions to Healthcare Costs" *Healthcare Finance News*. November, 2011.
14. Mello M, et al. "National Costs of the Medical Liability System." *Health Affairs*. 2010 Sep;29(9):1569-77
15. Jackson Healthcare. "A Costly Defense: Physicians Sound Off On The High Price of Defensive Medicine in the U.S." September, 2011. Accessed at: http://www.jacksonhealthcare.com/media/8968/defensivemedicine_ebook_final.pdf.

Chapter 26 References

1. Kocher R and Sahni N, Hospitals' Race to Employ Physicians-The Logic behind a Money-Losing Proposition. *NEJM* 364;19, 1790-1793.
2. Donald E. Konold, A Histroy of American Medical Ethics 1847-1912, at 14-16 (1962).
3. *Id.* at 22.
4. Nicole Huberfeld, *Be Not Afraid of Change: Time to Eliminate the Corporate Practice of Medicine Doctrine,* Health Matrix: Journal Of Law-Medicine. Vol 14, No. 2, 2004.
5. Michael Schaff and Glenn Prives. "The Corporate Practice of Medicine Doctrine: Is it Applicable to Your Client?" American Health Lawyers Association business Law and Governance Practice Group. Vol 3. Issue 2 May 2010. Available at: www.wilentz.com/files/articlesandpubliationfile/the%20corporate%20practice%20of%20medicine%20doctrine.pdf
6. To see the laws in your state go to http://www.aaem.org/corporatepractice/states.php
7. Mark A. Hall & Justin Vaugh, The Corporate Practice Of Medicine, Health Care Corporate Law: Formation And Regulation. Sec 3.4 at 3-14. (Mark A. Hall ed. 1999)
8. Andrew Ficher, Owning a Piece of the Doc: State Law Restraints on Lay Ownership of Healthcare Enterprises, *J. Health* L.39 (2006).
9. Committee On Quality Healthcare In America, Institute Of Medicine, Crossing The Quality Chasm: A New Health System For The 21st Century at 17-19 (2001).
10. See FICHER *supra* note 10.
11. Victoria Elliott. "ACOs, already surging, poised for even more growth," December, 2012 amednews.com at www.ama-assn.org/amednews/2012/12/10/bisc1210.htm.

Chapter 27 References

1. Centers for Disease Control. "Access to Trauma Centers in the United States." September 2009.
2. Mullins, RJ. A Historical Perspective of Trauma System Development in the United States. *The Journal of Trauma: Injury, Infection, and Critical Care*. 1999: 47(3); S8-S14.
3. Committee on Trauma and Committee on Shock, Division of Medical Sciences, National Academy of Sciences, National Research Council. Accidental Death and Disability: The Neglected Disease of Modern Society. The National Academies Press. 1966.
4. Illinois Department of Health. "31 Years Ago in IDPH History." http://www.idph.state.il.us/ webhistory20.htm. Accessed September 5, 2010.
5. American College of Surgeons Committee on Trauma. *Resources for Optimal Care of the Injured Patient*, 2006.
6. Bazzoli, GJ et al. Progress in the Development of Trauma Systems in the United States: Results of a National Survey. *JAMA*. 1995; 273(5): 395-401.
7. Mackenzie, EJ et al. A National Evaluation of the Effect of Trauma-Center Care on Mortality. *NEJM*. 2006; 354(4): 366-378.
8. Nathens, AB et al. The Effect of Organized Systems of Trauma Care on Motor Vehicle Crash Mortality. *JAMA*. 2000; 283(15): 1990-1994.
9. Mackenzie, EJ et al. National Inventory of Hospital Trauma Centers. JAMA. 2003; 289(12): 1515-1522.
10. Jauch E, et al. 2010 American Heart Association Guidelines for Cardiopulmonary Resuscitation and Emergency Cardiovascular Care Science, Part 11: Adult Stroke. *Circulation*. 2010; 122: S818-S828
11. Alberts MJ, et al. Recommendations for the Establishment of Primary Stroke Centers. *JAMA*. 2000;283(23):3102-3109.
12. The Joint Commission. Facts about Primary Stroke Center Certification. July 2012. Accessed at: http://www.jointcommission.org/assets/1/18/Facts_about_Primary_Stroke_ Center_Certification.pdf
13. Centers for Disease Control and Prevention. A summary of primary stroke center policy in the United States. Atlanta: U.S. Department of Health and Human Services; 2011.
14. Alberts, MJ et al. Special Report: Recommendations for Comprehensive Stroke Centers: A Consensus Statement From the Brain Attack Coalition. *Stroke*. 2005; 36: 1597-1616
15. The Joint Comission. Advanced Certification Comprehensive Stroke Centers. July 12, 2012. Accessed at: http://www.jointcommission.org/certification/advanced_certification_ comprehensive_stroke_centers.aspx
16. Anderson, HR et al. A Comparison of Coronary Angioplasty with Fibrinolytic Therapy in Acute Myocardial Infarction. *N Engl J Med*. 2003; 349:733-742
17. Concannon, TW et al. A Percutaneous Coronary Intervention Lab in Every Hospital? *Circulation: Cardiovascular Quality and Outcomes*. 2012; 5: 14-20
18. Jollis, JG et al. Systems of Care for ST-Segment–Elevation Myocardial Infarction: A Report From the American Heart Association's Mission: Lifeline. *Circulation: Cardiovascular Quality and Outcomes*. 2012; 5: 423-428
19. Krumholz, HR et al. Improvements in Door-to-Balloon Time in the United States, 2005 to 2010. *Circulation*. 2011; 124: 1038-1045
20. Jollis, JG et al. Expansion of a Regional ST-Segment–Elevation Myocardial Infarction System to an Entire State. *Circulation*. 2012; 126: 189-195
21. Granger, CB et al. Development of Systems of Care for ST-Elevation Myocardial Infarction Patients: The Primary Percutaneous Coronary Intervention (ST-Elevation Myocardial Infarction–Receiving) Hospital Perspective. *Circulation*. 2007; 116: e55-e59
22. Miedema, MD et al. Causes of Delay and Associated Mortality in Patients Transferred With ST-Segment–Elevation Myocardial Infarction. *Circulation*. 2011; 124: 1636-1644

23. Mathews R et al. Use of emergency medical service transport among patients with ST-segment-elevation myocardial infarction: findings from the National Cardiovascular Data Registry Acute Coronary Treatment Intervention Outcomes Network Registry-Get With The Guidelines. *Circulation.* 2011;124:154–63.

24. American College of Cardiology Foundation/American Heart Association Task Force on Practice Guidelines Writing Committee. 2013 ACCF/AHA Guideline for the Management of ST-Elevation Myocardial Infarction. *Circulation.* 2013; 127: e362-e425.

Chapter 28 References

1. See http://www.iep.utm.edu/ethics
2. See http://aspe.hhs.gov/admnsimp/pl104191.htm.
3. See http://www.hhs.gov/ocr/privacy/hipaa/understanding/summary/privacysummary. pdf.
4. See http://www.justice.gov/usao/eousa/foia_reading_room/usam/title9/131mcrm.htm
5. See http://uscode.house.gov/download/pls/18C63.txt
6. Hoffman L. House staff activism: the emergence of patient-care demands. *J Health Polit Policy Law.* 1982;7:421-439.
7. See http://www.emra.org/uploadedFiles/EMRA/About_EMRA/Representative_Council/Spring%202010%20CouncilSA%20REP%20HANDBOOK.pdf
8. American College of Emergency Physicians. Code of Ethics for Emergency Physicians. http://www.acep.org/practres.aspx?id=29144
9. American Medical Association. AMA Code of Medical Ethics, Opinion 9.025 – Advocacy for Change in Law and Policy.
10. American Medical Association. AMA Code of Medical Ethics, Opinion 9.025 – Advocacy for Change in Law and Policy.
11. ANA Code of Ethics. See: http://www.nursingworld.org/MainMenuCategories/EthicsStandards/CodeofEthicsforNurses/Code-of-Ethics.pdf
12. ANA Code Of Ethics ANA Code Of Ethics See: http://www.nursingworld.orgMainMenuCategories/EthicsStandards/CodeofEthicsforNurses/Code-of-Ethics.pdf
13. ENA Code Of Ethics. See http://www.ena.org/about/mission/Pages/Default.aspx.
14. Grey L. How to Win a Local Election. First M. Evans, 2007, 3rd Ed. p 31.

Chapter 29 References

1. Chassin, J & M Loeb. The Ongoing Quality Improvement Journey: Next Stop, High Reliability. *Health Affairs,* 30, no.4 (2011):559-568
2. Newhouse, Joseph P. (1993) Free for All? Lessons from the RAND Health Insurance Experiment. Harvard University Press, pg 173.
3. Institute of Medicine Report. Nov 1999. To Err is Human: Building A Safer Health System Available at http://www.iom.edu
4. Jha, A & D. Classen. Getting Moving on Patient Safety — Harnessing Electronic Data for Safer Care. *NEJM* 365;19 November0, 2011
5. Nelson et al. Prospective Trial of Real-Time Electronic Surveillance to Expedite Early Care of Severe Sepsis. *Annals of Emergency Medicine* Vol 57, No 5: May 2011
6. Ainsworth and Buchan. A tool for integrated care pathway variance analysis. *Stud Health Tecnol Inform* 2012; 180:995-999.
7. R Bohmer. The Four Habits of High-Value Health Care Organizations. *NEJM* 365;22 December, 2011

8. Matrix prioritization – based across multiple variables – exists in current ToDo software programs. Toodledo.com, as one example, accounts for the priority, importance, and deadline as separate independent factors for prioritization.

9. Atul Gawande. Big Med. *The New Yorker* August 13, 2012.

10. These can be recorded, or viewed on a closed circuit-style television. Including recording devices in ED resuscitation bays would have a real-time benefit to patient care. First, charting could be done accurately, without detracting from hands-on bedside care. Second, medical legal issues could be resolved through a review of concrete events as they were recorded.

11. J Frankovich et al. Evidence Based Medicine in the EMR Era. *NEJM* 365; 19 November, 2011

12. Benneyan et al. Statistical process control as a tool for research and healthcare improvement. *Qual Saf Health Care* 2003;12:458–464.

13. Scanning the horizon: emerging hospital-wide technologies and their impact on critical care. *Critical Care* February 2005 Vol 9 No 1 Suntharalingam *et al.*

14. Tenet example of prognostic scores to streamline admissions and hospital operations process: http://www.ahrq.gov/clinic/pneumonia/pneumonria.htm#pneumonia

15. Blumenthal — Wiring the Health System — Origins and Provisions of a New Federal Program *NEJM* 365;24 December 15, 2011

16. J Greene. Obama's $19 Billion book to Health Care IT: Mammoth Investment Fasttracks Electronic Health Records Annals of Emergency Medicine Vol 53; No. 5: May 2009